Inspired Physician Leadership

Creating influence and impact

By Charles R. Stoner and Jason S. Stoner

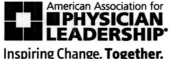

American Association for
PHYSICIAN
LEADERSHIP
Inspiring Change. **Together.**

Toll-free: 800-562-8088
Fax: 813-287-8993
Web: physicianleaders.org
Email: info@physicianleaders.org

400 N. Ashley Drive, Suite 400 • Tampa, Florida 33602-4322

ISBN: 978-0-924674-05-1

Library of Congress Card Number: 2015945450

Printed in the United States of America by Lightning Source.

iii

Prologue
Physician Leadership:
Transitions and Challenges

WE ARE BEHAVIORISTS, NOT CLINICIANS. OUR RESEARCH, WRITing, and consulting centers on leadership and explores the complex set of interpersonal dynamics that live as the heart and soul of meaningful, difference-making, authentic leadership.

Over the past twenty years, our work has taken us into large health care systems, regional hospitals, specialty centers and private practices. We work, often one-on-one, with talented physicians — observing; listening; coaching; at times, advising; and constantly amazed at and grateful for the receptivity extended. Yet, we are always cognizant that while we have been allowed the privilege of touching your world, we are outsiders. This project began because of physicians who prompted us (or challenged us) to extend our interpersonal behavioral applications to the realm of physician leadership. And, this book was born.

Inspired Physician Leadership is guided by two central tenets. First, physicians deal with evidence. You favor clear data and solid research over conjecture and experience-based, anecdotal approaches. As such, any book on physician leadership must be grounded in sound research, accepted theory and informed best practices. Such is our intent.

Second, since physicians are intensely busy, the delivery must be practical, realistic and approachable. The book must address key issues and offer workable solutions to real concerns and situations that physicians encounter. In short, you demand an engaging blend of evidence and pragmatism. We have strived, first and foremost, to achieve this blend of a compelling and engaging read. The field of interpersonal behavior and leadership has a rich

and highly applicable base of understanding that is both relevant and needed by a physician leader audience. *Inspired Physician Leadership* is based
on clear and applicable evidence that is presented with dynamic relevancy.

There is one final caveat, of sorts. Most books in this field take a broad,
encompassing, and rather tactical approach — covering an array of themes
ranging from budgeting to staffing to strategizing to dealing with people.
As such, these works often miss the importance of a deep behavioral understanding and finesse that comes from a careful grounding in the interpersonal and contextual dynamics at play. It is not our intention to be a one-stop,
mini-MBA for physicians. Without apology, *Inspired Physician Leadership*
focuses on the physician's personal transition into the realm of leadership
and the interpersonal challenges that accompany this new, expanded, and
largely unfamiliar role.

Dozens of physician leaders at various career stages and levels have offered insight and perspective over the course of this project. We are grateful
for their time, their patience and their willingness to help us make this book
as relevant as possible. In particular, we must extend a special thanks to Dr.
Matthew Scott for being both a friend and a reflective sounding board. In
most cases, throughout the book, individual names have been changed and
situations may be altered slightly to maintain the dynamics of the example
while protecting identities. In a few cases, composite examples have been used.

A special thanks must be extended to Bill Steiger of the American Association for Physician Leadership®. Bill has been a keen editor who has offered
guidance, rapid response to our queries and a careful eye on the changing
world of physician leadership.

Finally, yet foremost, this book is dedicated to an amazing scholar, thought
leader, wife and mom — Dr. Julie Stoner.

Contents

....

1

Today: The Case for Physician Leadership

....

CONTEMPORARY HEALTH CARE ORGANIZATIONS ARE ENGAGED IN unprecedented transformational change. Although clarity is masked, the future will yield new and challenging models of practice and delivery. Like all transformational changes, disruption abounds as traditional assumptions and approaches bend to the winds of powerful economic, social, political and demographic pressures.

While the future of health care remains problematic, experts agree that physician leaders must be at the table, engaged as principal players among those who will define and shape tomorrow's health care strategies.[1] Beyond the considerations of broad strategy and policy, a range of fundamental and immediate factors demand attention. As such, the call for physician leadership arises within a context of competing needs — expanding health care demands, systemwide motives for efficiency and questions about our capacity to respond while maintaining patient-centrality with sound clinical outcomes.

The gravity and complexity of these overlapping needs lead experts to conclude that the emphasis on clinical leadership is an essential reality rather than the latest passing fancy.[2] Increasingly, expert voices declare that "the leadership needed to transform the performance of hospitals and health care systems must come primarily from doctors and other clinicians."[3]

The Need for Physician Leadership

The need for physician leadership has never been more critical. We begin by considering three reasons. The first, drawn from the insightful work of

Harvard professor Richard Bohmer, resonates deeply with clinicians.

Bohmer argues that as health care reform intensifies, physician leaders help assure that patient well-being will not become a subservient concern in the face of politically charged issues of cost containment and revised delivery models.[4] Physician leaders appear to be our best choice for ensuring that these complicated decisions will be firmly grounded in health care's central mission of patient care and outcomes.

There is no escaping bottom-line reality. Health care organizations face far-reaching challenges that demand "increasingly difficult tradeoffs ... (that) balance the allocation of scarce resources to individual patient care and the care of communities and populations."[5] Medical leaders are best suited to understand and make these tradeoffs.[6] Expanding this theme, experts argue that physicians, with their training and practice, bring a mindset of clinical realism that is fundamental when grappling with these tough choices. In short, physician leaders possess "a deep intuitive knowledge about the core business ... that helps with decision-making and institutional strategy."[7]

The second reason physician leadership is needed is more nuanced — imbued with deep behavioral themes. Physician leaders, because of their acquired levels of expertise and credibility, are poised to be key mediators between practicing physicians and the organization's non-clinical leadership.[8] As potential conduits of understanding, physician leaders can influence an array of interdependent constituencies who may have difficulty envisioning perspectives beyond their own. Of course, this potential is achieved only when physician leaders successfully navigate the tricky maze of interpersonal and politically charged dynamics that make impactful leadership so challenging.

The third reason has been the subject of extensive and spirited debated. A growing array of experts, however, believes that when doctors are engaged in maintaining and enhancing organizational performance, better financial and clinical outcomes occur.[9]

In one of the few empirical investigations of its type, Amanda Goodall examined hospital performance outcomes according to CEO classification — either physician leaders or non-physician leaders. Data were collected from 100 U.S. hospitals (each with top-level rankings) and included 300 CEOs. Quality outcomes were assessed in three specialty areas: cancer, digestive disorders and heart surgery. The study found a strong positive association between physician leadership and hospital quality rankings.[10]

Notwithstanding some obvious methodological constraints inherent in such data, at least three important conclusions can be drawn. First, as noted earlier, physician leaders may experience a success differential because they have a deeper understanding of core clinical dynamics than their non-clinical counterparts do. Second, physician leaders have developed strong connections with the medical staff that should yield important advantages — an understanding ear and informed voice, competency-based trust and clinical credibility. Third, physician credibility pays dividends in many tangential areas, including the likelihood of attracting talented medical professionals to their organizations.[11]

In the face of such powerful rationale, the call for physician leadership places us squarely on the horns of a dilemma. While the need for physician leaders is apparent and growing, an insufficient number are poised to engage and succeed in leadership roles. Physicians stepping into new roles as organizational leaders are often underprepared to thrive in this new context. Although medical schools are increasingly adding some leadership components to their courses of study, there remains little in the physicians' formal training that prepares them for positions of leadership.[12] In fact, a recent report drew the dramatic conclusion that "despite evidence supporting the link between leadership and improved clinical outcomes, a significant frontline leadership gap exists in health care."[13]

Any discussion of the rationale for physician leadership must address an additional complication: Experts predict a national shortage of an estimated 90,000 physicians by 2020 and 130,000 by 2025.[14] Jeff Cain, MD, president of the American Academy of Family Physicians, noted a confluence of factors that have dramatically affected the demand for services. Our population is growing and aging — two factors that signal increased health care needs. Against this demographic backdrop, add the impact of the Affordable Care Act, which could account for 30 million newly insured individuals seeking primary care.[15]

There is a further complication. The number of new physicians entering the workforce each year has not grown appreciably in the past 20 years. Compounding this depletion, evidence indicates that practicing doctors are likely to retire earlier than previously anticipated. In fact, the Association of American Medical Colleges has estimated that nearly one-third of all physicians — approximately 250,000 — will retire by 2020.[16]

In general, physicians have been reluctant or ambivalent about assuming formal leadership roles.[17] Scholars have suggested at least three reasons for this hesitancy: financial disincentives, status disincentives and training and skill deficiencies.[18] Regarding the latter point, some observers have boldly asserted that "there is nothing in a physician's education and training that qualifies him (or her) to be a leader."[19]

What does all this mean for our purposes? As in any situation where demand for services significantly outstrips the supply of talent, we must be careful in the deployment of our talent resources or risk exacerbating the problem. Leadership roles reduce a physician's time in direct clinical care. As such, we must identify physicians who appear to possess both clinical expertise and strong potential for leadership success. Further, we must help this cadre of promising physician leaders develop the perspectives, mindset and skills (the bulk of which can broadly be classified as interpersonal in nature) to meet the challenges of leadership with insight, authenticity, confidence and impact.

Arguably, the selection and development of high-potential physician leaders may be one of the most critical challenges facing our health care organizations. Drawing from leadership pioneer Jim Collins, part of this challenge will be making sure that we get the right people in the right spots.[20]

Accepting the mantle of leadership, one encounters a landscape that is familiar in nature but strange in complexity. As we will discuss in the next few chapters, the transition from clinician to clinician leader is behaviorally nuanced and interpersonally intense. And evidence suggests that many physician leaders recognize a formidable gap between the well-honed expertise they possess and the toolkit needed for leadership success.[21] The focus of this book is to close that gap. Importantly, we accept that leadership is "an observable, understandable, learnable set of skills and practices" — an arena capable of enhancement and development.[22] Before progressing, however, a deeper understanding of the nature of contemporary leadership is in order.

The Nature of Leadership

In a recent review of clinical leadership, researchers suggested that the "widespread fascination with leadership may be because it is such a mysterious process."[23] Echoing this thought, leadership pioneer Bernard Bass has noted that "there are almost as many different definitions of leadership as there are persons who have attempted to define the concept."[24] Indeed. Rather than offer an easily forgotten, all-encompassing sweep, we have chosen to target just a few of the more powerful explanatory attempts.

In refreshingly succinct fashion, best-selling scholar Peter Senge suggested that leaders "inspire" others.[25] There is deep insight and significance to this perspective. Consider the etymology of the word inspire, suggesting that one who inspires "breathes life into" others. Daniel Goleman, Richard Boyatzis and Annie McKee extended this framing, indicating that "Great leaders ... ignite our passions and inspire the best in us."[26]

Apparent in these two definitions is the realization that leadership plays an "expansive role" when it is successful. Indeed, effective leaders have the capacity to bring out the best in others. In our phrasing, impactful leaders "unleash the talent in others so their full potential can be realized."

Have you ever been to a Bruce Springsteen concert? Whether you are a diehard fan or a take-it-or-leave-it observer, there is no escaping the power of the event. For nearly four hours, the drumbeat never stops and Springsteen never leaves the stage as the E Street Band pours every ounce of raw emotion and energy into the performance. Now here is the key. Members of the E Street Band, each distinguished musicians in their own right, will tell you the same thing. They perform at their very best when they are with Springsteen. That is the image and tone of leadership that is needed — engaging the talent around us so others can perform and contribute at the top of their game.

There is a second key theme. Leaders create and exert influence. This concept of influence is both intentional and directed. In essence, leaders create influence that "touches the feelings, emotions, thinking and actions of others so that goals and visions are realized."[27] The idea that leadership encapsulates the capacity to create intentional influence is a multilayered process that we will refine in later chapters.

Let's add another timely perspective. In a classic work, Harvard professor John Kotter argued that leaders "cope with change."[28] In this regard, he emphasized three fundamental functions of leadership: establishing direction, aligning people and motivating and inspiring. This forward-looking approach is relevant for all competitive organizations, and speaks to the turbulent reshaping that frames our contemporary health care environment.

Yet Kotter's version of leadership is often misunderstood. A colleague once opined, with only minimal sarcasm, that "administrators manage chaos, and leaders create it." The latter phrase is dangerously repugnant. In fact, the finesse of leadership comes in the capacity to move people, teams and organizations to embrace change precisely without the experience of chaos. The ways to achieve this intricately balanced outcome serve as the foundations of this book.

Finally, we encourage you to consider a broad view of leadership. We are long past the days when leadership was compartmentalized, the purview of a select few perched at the top of an organization's hierarchy. Leaders, some with formal designations and some without (informal leaders), are scattered throughout our organizations. When formal leaders misunderstand or minimize the influence that is wielded by their informal counterparts, both efficiencies and effectiveness are at risk.

Many of you, drawing from the credibility of your clinical backgrounds and the strength of your personalities, wield influence that belies any formal position or title. At times, informal leadership allows one the freedom and flexibility to behave in ways that may be blocked to those holding formal positions that require stricter adherence to the "company line." While this book focuses on the challenges of formal leadership, the concepts we present have merit for those of you who seek to expand your influence through more informal means.

The Differential Impact of Leadership

Transparency demands that we address a question that philosophically frames all that follows. It is the question of leader impact — a question that has spawned years of debate and pointed controversy. The controversy is not whether leadership matters but the extent. In short, how much does leadership really matter? What is the differential impact of leadership?

As with most complex issues, experts fail to display complete agreement. Some scholars cynically opine that even our most talented leaders have minimal impact on overall organizational performance. Instead, these critics argue, key external or environmental factors — such as spikes and declines in the economy, shifting patterns of client and market expectations, industry transitions and sociopolitical trends — are far more critical drivers of performance than leadership acumen.[29]

Despite these arguments, the preponderance of evidence over the last two decades has presented a different view. Researchers, scholars and thought leaders have argued that leadership plays a significant role in performance, as well as a range of other positive organizational outcomes (such as trust, culture and the overall interpersonal dynamics of the workplace).[30]

For example, consider a specialty clinic that in the past two years has seen three of its heavily recruited and brightest young stars leave the practice. Such turnover is not only costly but ripples throughout the clinic, affecting colleagues, staff and patients, as well as the overall image of the clinic. While we certainly do not know all the factors rumbling behind this turnover, we can comfortably argue that our immediate leaders have a dramatic impact on the way we experience and feel about our work.

The Physician Leader

Physician leadership or clinical leadership is a broad term, largely because of the range of roles that may be included and the array of paths that may be pursued. Leadership in the clinical realm is certainly among the most idiosyncratic of any industry. Broad generalizations diminish the complexity of roles that physician leaders hold. Further, physician leadership usually involves a mix of clinically based and administratively based roles. With this in mind, researchers have identified three types of clinical leaders: institutional leaders, service leaders —such as department chairs or research directors — and frontline leaders, those who are serve as a key point of contact with direct patient care and are responsible for clinical outcomes.[31]

Although intensity varies with each of these roles, a shift is apparent. While our clinical activities focus on decision-making at the individual physician/patient level, "leadership necessarily involves stepping away from the individual physician/patient relationship and examining problems at a systems level, requiring the ability to view issues broadly and systematically."[32]

Physician leaders are people like Matthew Gorman, who spends part of his time devoted to his private practice in internal medicine, work that highlights the excitement and meaning of direct patient care. Referring to his practice, Gorman's words echo what many of you no doubt believe: "This is why I became a doctor in the first place."

Increasingly, however, Gorman has been asked to assume leadership roles within his health care organization. Currently, he serves as director of informatics. He works with an assortment of high-profile project teams — often as the sole physician — to address critical quality and patient service initiatives. These systemwide leadership activities put Gorman at the cutting edge, helping to shape the future.

Physician leaders are also people like Ronald Lander, chairman of the department of neurosurgery at a major university. A respected neurosurgeon, Lander finds energy and excitement in a range of leadership roles. Armed with an MBA, he can address both business and clinical exchanges with insight and perspective. He enjoys working on important, difference-making initiatives because he knows that he possesses unique skills that help "move the needle forward." He also mentors younger physicians and helps to create and maintain a world-class department. Further, Lander's blend of experience and perspective has led to his inclusion in key professional associations, as well as community and service activities, bringing his leadership into a broader social arena.

Moving into physician leadership requires that you embrace a "leadership mindset," which is different from the traditional "clinical mindset." We view this change as a developmental transition, and that transition will be the focus of the next chapter. In addition, you must master a set of interpersonal skills that may be unfamiliar, underdeveloped or underused. Again, these will be discussed throughout our subsequent chapters.

Here, a key question must be posed — fortunately one that has been the focus of considerable research, as well as a range of informed and thoughtful discourse. What competencies do high-potential physician leaders really need? Let's look at the data.

Drawing from interviews with faculty physicians at the Cleveland Clinic, researchers found four recurring themes that were seen as requisite for physicians aspiring to leadership positions. The themes: position-related knowledge of finance, budgets, etc., and field-related expertise; people skills, including dimensions of emotional intelligence; vision, and organizational orientation, including understanding the history and operating structure of the organization and a commitment to working for the good of the organization.[33] Importantly, within the context of this study, the people-oriented and emotional intelligence theme was most frequently noted.

Numerous studies have specified the more critical of these leadership skills and competencies, portraying a decidedly behavioral perspective. With remarkable consistency, studies have a noted several interpersonal factors. These include engaging in deep listening and respectful communication, generating persuasive arguments and creating influence and buy-in, demonstrating conflict resolution and negotiation, applying emotional and social intelligence, understanding teamwork and team building, understanding and working effectively in politicized contexts, providing vision, motivating others, and leading transformational change.[34] Attention to these critical interpersonal factors provides the framework of this book.

Performance Clarity Through Crystal-Clear Expectations

Although our exploration of leadership will have a decidedly behavioral thrust, we must conclude this opening chapter by underscoring the centrality of performance and crystal-clear expectations.

Performance is the unmitigated, essential metric of leadership. In his No. 1 bestseller, *Good to Great,* Harvard professor Jim Collins differentiated highly successful leaders from others. Among his major findings were that these top-level leaders demonstrated an unwavering focus on performance.[35]

We will highlight throughout this book the importance of setting and carefully communicating crystal-clear expectations. There are few themes of greater significance. Scholars have studied the nature of performance expectations, and we accept that performance is enhanced when expectations are clear, specific and challenging.[36] The behavioral dynamics underlying these criteria are well established and help us avoid the toxic lure of "do-your-best" goals. When performance targets are missed and when questionable and problematic behaviors surface, we always return to the mantra of clarifying expectations.

Physicians certainly understand the prominence of high standards and challenging expectations. Excellence is paramount and mistakes are abhorred, largely because of the risks involved. However, assuring that others recognize and understand these expectations may be an area begging for greater attention. Physicians, being quick studies with high personal standards, readily accept demanding standards of performance and assume that others respond similarly and are onboard. This can result in disappointment and frustration as others fail to grasp the level of performance needed. State and restate your expectations — crystal-clear expectations — as a starting point. High, challenging, uncompromised performance expectations are keys to success.

We see important links between our attention to interpersonal dynamics and performance. Understanding behavioral complexities and nuance will enhance the interpersonal context, unleashing the potential and talent of all involved, and thereby helping to ensure immediate and longer-term performance. Further, as standards of performance change — as they assuredly will in the turbulent world of health care — the behavioral tone you have established will help you adapt nimbly and less disruptively.

Concluding Thoughts: The Leader as Trailblazer

Leaders are trailblazers. They always have been. Some members of your organization — be it a professional office practice, specialty clinic, regional hospital or massive health care system — are comfortable with clearly defined and segmented roles that can be executed with precision and quality. These "diligent doers" are the heart and soul of action — the proverbial "good citizens" of collective organizational life.

Still others are natural administrators, capable of bringing structure and order to seeming confusion. They assign tasks, administer budgets and align resources to meet target goals. They are careful and judicious caretakers who assure effectiveness and efficiency around our central missions. They ensure that care is provided within a context of limited resources.

But you are different. You do not eschew these foundational roles, and you have, in all likelihood, demonstrated considerable proficiency as one who performs your clinical duties with competence. Moving into the challenges of leadership, you remain a respected and reliable font of clinical expertise and wisdom. Yet there is more.

As we have noted, it will be your job to challenge systemic status quo; to urge and move others to new frontiers. And, as we will see shortly, you must push these frontiers while others bask in relative comfort and security. Unlike your peers, you transcend "what is" and veer into the nebulous territory of "what can be" and "what should be" and "what must be."

If you are a leader, you have the rare and elusive capacity to embrace others, understand their condition, move fearlessly into the realm of emotional understanding, capture the minds and hearts of others and unleash their talents. As you push the boundaries of progress, you bring others with you. You understand the reality, perhaps even the essential contradiction of leadership — we succeed through others. Leadership failures are rarely because of a dearth of good ideas, insightful visions and competitively accurate strategies. Leaders fail because they cannot traverse the behavioral complexity and interpersonal nuance of emboldening others to embrace the journey.

Previews of Coming Attractions

Although the need for physician leaders has received considerable attention, there has been limited focus on what doctors must actually do to become difference-making leaders.[37] Our goal is to facilitate that focus through a careful, in-depth plunge into the critical behavioral and interpersonal dynamics that undergird contemporary leadership. As such, let's offer a brief overview of subsequent chapters.

In Chapter 2, "Transitions: The Nature and Challenge of Clinician/Leader Interplay," we will explore the dynamics and complexities of the various forms of clinician/leader roles and the transitions that these roles present. Chapter 3, "Tone: The Significance of the Interpersonal Factor," builds the case, through data and example, that the leader's interpersonal awareness and finesse can be a key foundation for success. Elements of emotional intelligence will be woven throughout the chapter. Importantly, this chapter introduces a series of interpersonal themes and considerations that represent new ways of looking at people and generating desired outcomes.

In Chapter 4, "Dialogue: Communicating for Understanding and Influence," we provide a unique look at creating reciprocal understanding through deep listening, respectful inquiry, open-ended questioning and engaged dialogue. We put these ideas into bottom-line practices, emphasizing clear communication and the ongoing use of "brief coaching encounters."

Chapter 5 explores the theme of "Teamwork: The Foundations of Collective Synergy." Physicians are used to working in teams. In fact, the operating room may be one of the most finely honed conceptualizations of teamwork in action that we could ever find. However, surgical teams differ dramatically from project and administrative teams that physician leaders now encounter. This pivotal chapter deals with key team issues that may be new for physician leaders. Drawing from solid research and theory, this chapter presents a practical set of skills and competencies.

Chapter 6 addresses the ever-relevant theme of "Conflict: The Power of Respectful Conflict Encounters." Research has consistently placed conflict (and more specifically how to respectfully and successfully address conflict) as one of the major concerns and stumbling blocks for leaders. This chapter explores how conflict arises and evolves, and we discuss how to address tough, interpersonal conflict.

In Chapter 7, "Negotiations: Politics and Principled Outcomes," we explore the array of political dynamics that often frustrate physician leaders. Armed with this perspective, we address the dynamics of negotiating and the importance of the understanding and judicious use of influence.

Chapter 8 addresses the timely and critical themes of "Motivation: Building Performance Through People." This chapter will help you understand how you can build a sense of commitment and engagement where people experience challenge, energy, fulfillment and ownership. Proven approaches drawn from underlying theory are examined.

Chapter 9, "Change: A Future of Opportunity," will challenge your thinking about and approach to change. We next explore the very real and common pitfall of initiative decay and address how leaders can mitigate its impact. We offer a model of change, which draws heavily on the behavioral and interpersonal topics discussed throughout the book. Finally, Chapter 10, "Tomorrow: A Case for Possibility," offers a brief view of the resilience needed for physician leaders to move forward as key difference-makers in health care's future.

---

1. Mountford, J. & Webb, C. (2009). Clinical leadership: Unlocking high performance in healthcare. London: McKinsey. Schwartz, R.W. & Pogge, C. (2000). Physician leadership: Essential skills in a changing environment. *The American Journal of Surgery, 180*(3), 187-192.

2. Darzi, A. (2009). A time for revolutions: The role of clinicians in health care reform. *New England Journal of Medicine, 361*(6), e8.

3. Mountford, J. & Webb, C. (2009). When clinicians lead. *McKinsey Quarterly,* February, p. 1.

4. Bohmer, R. (2012). *The instrumental value of medical leadership: Engaging doctors in improving services.* The King's Fund.

5. Bohmer, 2012, p. 6.

6. Ibid.

7. Goodall, A.H. (2011). Physician leaders and hospital performance: Is there an association? *Social Science & Medicine, 73,* 535-539, p. 538.

8. Falcone, R.E. & Satiani, B. (2008). Physician as hospital chief executive officer. *Vascular and Endovascular Surgery, 42,* 88-94. Guthrie, 1999.

9. Dwyer, A.J. (2010). Medical managers in contemporary healthcare organizations: A consideration of the literature. *Australian Health Review, 34,* 514-522. Falcone, B.E. & Satiani, B. (2008). Physician as hospital chief executive officer. *Vascular and Endovascular Surgery, 42,* 88-94. Stoller, J.K. (2009). Developing physician-leaders: A call to action. *Journal of General Internal Medicine, 24,* 876-878.

10. Goodall, 2011.

11. Falcone & Satiani, 2008.

12. Snell, A.J.; Briscoe, D.; & Dickson, G. (2011). From the inside out: The engagement of physicians as leaders in health care settings. *Qualitative Health Research, 21*(7), 952-967. Stephenson, J. (2009). Getting down to business. *Management of Health Care, 339,* 1170-1171.

13. Blumenthal, D.M.; Bernard, K.; Bohnen, J.; & Bohmer, R. (2012). Addressing the leadership gap in medicine: Residents' need for systematic leadership development training. *Academic Medicine, 87*(4), 513-522.

14. Angle, J. (2013). Retiring doctors mean problems for newly insured under ObamaCare. **www.foxnews.com/politics/2013/08/26/retiring**; retrieved December 10, 2014.

15. Ibid.

16. Albert, M. (2011). Warnings of doctor shortage go unheeded. **http://remappingdebate. org/article/warnings-doctor-shortage-go-unheeded**.

17. Bohmer, 2012.

18. Mountford, J. & Webb, C. (2009) When clinicians lead. *McKinsey Quarterly,* February.

19. Ibid., p. 68.

20. Collins, J. (2001). *Good to Great: Why some companies make the leap ... and others don't.* New York: HarperCollins.

21. Blumenthal, Bernard, Bohnen, & Bohmer, 2012.

22. Kouzes, J.M. (1998). Finding your voice. In L.C. Spears (Ed.). *Insights on Leadership: Service, stewardship, spirit, and servant-leadership* (pp. 322-325). New York: John Wiley & Sons, p. 322.

23. Howieson, B. & Thiagarajah, T. (2011). What is clinical leadership? A journal-based meta-review. *The International Journal of Clinical Leadership, 17,* 7-18.

24. Bass, B.M. (2007). Concepts of leadership. In Vecchio, R.P. (ed.), *Leadership: Understanding the dynamics of power and influence in organizations* (2nd ed.), Notre Dame, IN: Notre Dame Press, 3-22, p. 16.

25. Senge, P.M. (2006). *The Fifth Discipline: The art and practice of the learning organization.* New York: Knopf.

26. Goleman, D.; Boyatzis, R.; & McKee, A. (2002). *Primal Leadership: Realizing the power of emotional intelligence.* Cambridge, MA: Harvard Business School Press.

27. Stoner, C.R. & Stoner, J.S. (2013). *Building Leaders: Paving the path for emerging leaders.* New York: Routledge, p. 4.

28. Kotter, J.P. (2001). What leaders really do. *Harvard Business Review, 79*(11), 85-96.

29. Pfeffer, J. (1977). The ambiguity of leadership. *Academy of Management Review, 2*(1), 104-112. Thomas, A.B. (1988). Does leadership make a difference to organizational performance? *Administrative Science Quarterly, 33,* 388-400.

30. Bass, B.M.; Avolio, B.J.; Jung, D.I.; & Berson, Y. (2003). Predicting unit performance by assessing transformational and transactional leadership. *Journal of Applied Psychology, 88*(2), 207-218. Judge, T.A.; Piccolo, R.F.; & Illies, R. (2004). The unforgotten one? The validity of consideration and initiating structure in leadership research. *Journal of Applied Psychology, 89*(1), 36-51.

31. Blumenthal, D.M.; Bernard, K.; Bohnen, J.; & Bohmer, R. (2012). Addressing the leadership gap in medicine: Residents' need for systematic leadership development training. *Academic Medicine, 87*(4), 513-522.

32. Collins-Nakai, R. (2006). Leadership in medicine. *McGill Journal of Medicine, 9,* 68-63, p. 68.

33. Taylor, C.A.; Taylor, J.C.; & Stoller, J.K. (2008). Exploring leadership competencies in established and aspiring physician leaders: An interview-based study. *Journal of General Internal Medicine, 23*(6), 748-754.

34. Ciampi, E.J.; Hunt, A.A.; Arenson, K.O.; Mordes, D.A.; Oldham, W.M.; Woo, K.V.; Owens, D.A.; Cannon, M.D.; & Dermody, T.S. (2011). A workshop on leadership for MD/PhD students. *Medical Education Online, 16*(7075), 1-9. McKenna, M.K.; Gartland, M.P.; & Pugno, P.A. (2004). Development of physician leadership competencies: Perceptions of physician leaders, physician educators, and medical students. *Journal of Health Administration Education, 21,* 343-354. Santric Milicevic, M.M; Bjegovic-Mikanovic, V.M.; Terzic-Supic, Z.J.; & Vasic, V. (2011). Competencies gap of management teams in primary health care. *European Journal of Public Health, 21,* 247-253. Taylor, C.A.; Taylor, J.C.; & Stoller, J.K. (2008). Exploring leadership competencies in established and aspiring physician leaders: An interview-based study. *Journal of General Internal Medicine, 23,* 748-754.

35. Collins, 2001.

36. Locke, E.A. & Latham, G.P. (2002). Building a practically useful theory of goal-setting and task motivation: A 35-year odyssey. *American Psychologist, 57*(9), 705-717.

37. Bohmer, p. 15.

2

Transitions: The Nature and Challenge
of Clinician/Leader Interplay

N THE PREVIOUS CHAPTER, WE ADDRESSED THE KEY QUESTION OF
what it means to lead. We envisioned physician leadership as an encompassing term that covered a range of clinician/leader interactions, roles and
challenges. We suggested that the expectations of physician leaders can become
quite nuanced and differ across varied contexts.

Importantly, we argued that contemporary physician leaders must move
beyond traditional role expectations, becoming more than detail-focused
administrators or messengers who feel charged to fight battles, secure resources and remove perceived obstacles for the clinicians they represent.[1] Of
course, leaders carry the representational voice of others, but they must do
more within our era of health care turbulence and ongoing change.

Progressive physician leaders must consider broad and at times competing perspectives. They must be able to listen with patience and reflection.
They must engage in the complex processes of dialogue, negotiation and
persuasion. They must embrace with agility the highly politicized process
of creating influence.

They must be able to work collectively with others as members of extended,
cross-disciplinary teams. They must be able to align people whose agendas
vary and build commitment. The chapters that follow represent a deep dive
into the more critical interpersonal and behavioral skills, competencies,
interactive approaches and activities needed to make difference-making
leadership come alive.

But this chapter is different. This chapter focuses on you and the transitional
nature of your move into physician leadership. As such, the chapter represents a

critical and often overlooked link between our broad introduction to leadership and the pragmatic behavioral themes that comprise the bulk of this book.

Why Lead?

Generally, three reasons prompt physicians to move from purely clinical roles into more expanded leadership roles. These reasons are not independent, and all may be drivers in the leadership decision. To explore these motivational drivers, we will introduce two physician leaders with whom we have recently worked.

Jim Grant is a respected surgeon with a track record of clinical successes. Turning 50, he began to feel the tug for more — new challenges, new opportunities, new ways to stretch and grow. Grant also knew that he had the capacity to get things done, and he enjoyed the challenge of accomplishing what others thought was nearly impossible. For Grant, leadership was a chance to extend his growth and use his considerable talents in new, expanded and creative roles. Reducing his clinical time, Grant jumped into leadership roles and guided some important and high-profile projects for his organization, and he participated as a team member on a groundbreaking innovation initiative. To Grant's thinking, he had always been a leader, and his new roles were simply part of his personal growth and development.

The first reason for gravitating toward leadership emerges from one's career progression. At some point, certain physicians, such as Grant, begin to look for new challenges and opportunities. Here, physicians may desire more strategic decision-making roles within their health care organizations. Or they may desire an opportunity to create broader impact, whether within a department, practice or larger hospital setting. Whatever the situation, physicians begin to curb direct clinical time and assume leadership roles.

In most cases, physicians take on blended or mixed roles — spending part of their time on traditional clinical duties and part of their time on new leadership duties.[2] Typically, these moves occur selectively and incrementally. In a pure sense, this decision is a result of one's "perception of contribution" — that is, the belief that a greater and more fulfilling contribution can be made to the organization and the profession by engaging in leadership activities.

Importantly, this move into leadership likely has payoffs to all parties involved. The organization and its members gain valuable perspective and guidance from talented physicians. In turn, physicians gain a deeper sense of fulfillment and significance that emanates from the realization that their influence is being felt on a more expanded scale. The challenge and energizing nature of taking on new activities are reasonable extensions of the physician's need for achievement.[3]

The second reason generally works in conjunction with the first. Consider the example of Regina Mills, a talented 42-year-old family practice physician who caught the attention of senior leaders within her health care system. Known for her intelligence, clinical savvy, calm demeanor and outstanding ability to communicate with patients and clinical staff, Mills was tabbed early and often to serve on committees and project teams for her parent organization. Flourishing in these new roles, she was asked to assume expanded leadership activities, eventuating into a key director's position emphasizing the quality of patient care.

As we see with Mills, physicians are often asked by senior organizational leaders to assume leadership roles. Generally, this request is based on proven clinical talents rather than a demonstrated aptitude for leadership.[4] In short, individual excellence, as evidenced through clinical success, serves as the prompt to organizational leaders that a given physician possesses strengths and perspectives that warrant broader opportunities for input and influence. In this regard, the physician's career progression follows a pattern similar to that of other professions — namely, promoting one to new roles based on achievement in previous roles.

There is considerable logic to this approach. Indeed, past success may be the most tangible criterion we possess for judging likelihood of success in expanded roles, and such decisions have the ring of fairness.[5] In addition, the talented and respected clinician carries considerable sway for enhancing the quality and acceptance of important organizational decisions. Commonly, as is the case with Mills, senior leaders see some evidence — albeit limited — that the physician has certain qualities that should enable success. Senior leaders intuit that key physicians must have a "seat at the table" and be included as progressive strategies and actions are considered. All of this reasoning is wrapped in the assumption of "transferability" — assuming that proven excellence in one highly challenging role (physician) can be extended into other highly challenging roles (various leadership assignments).

The third reason for stepping into a leadership role can be problematic, but is a factor that we encounter in a number of situations. Here, physicians assume tasks and responsibilities of leadership because no one else will do so — or, at least, no one else with any degree of leadership acumen is willing to do so. At times, drawing from a sense of presumed rotational logic, a physician may even matter-of-factly say, "I guess it's my turn to step into the role." Hopefully, even when prompted by this need or gap in service, physicians can experience the outcomes of added significance and contribution noted above.

Regardless of the reason or reasons, one thing is clear. Moving from successful clinician to difference-making leader represents a huge transition. Now, physician leaders must work in a more collective context, where their clinical expertise is appreciated but is insufficient for gaining support and action. Not surprisingly, physician leaders often find such non-clinical settings to be frustrating and difficult.

Key Transitions

Moving into the roles and responsibilities of physician leadership represents a personal and career transition — an evolutionary, somewhat natural and developmentally progressing movement. Yet the physician leadership transition can be profoundly nuanced and confusing. Consider the expressive way that Herminia Ibarra and others shape our thinking, as they describe transition as "a process of leaving one thing, without having fully left it, and at the same time entering something else, without fully being a part of it."[6] And so it is with the physician leader — clinician and leader — working to "straddle both worlds at the same time."[7]

Although one may assume that doctors are natural leaders, the claim may need to be tempered.[8] Consistent with most professions, some physicians have a stronger proclivity toward thinking and acting as leaders than do others. Similar to those coming from other technical arenas that demand high levels of specialized proficiency, the skills and competencies of leadership typically have not been part of the physician's training.[9] While this appears to be changing to some extent, physicians, especially younger ones, are often advised to protect their autonomy and avoid the lure of administrative and managerial duties.[10] In fact, leadership responsibilities have long been viewed as a "necessary evil" that comes with seniority.[11]

In the following sections, we will explore four important transitions that physicians generally encounter as they become physician leaders. Certainly, the nature and extent of these transitions are as idiosyncratic as are the individual physicians in our audience. However, all four transitions will, in some measure, be part of the physician leader's journey.

The Transition From Doer to Leader

Stepping into leadership evokes what many consider the most challenging career transition of all — the transition from being a "doer" who achieves success by depending on oneself and the strength of personal performance to being a "leader" who achieves success (at least in part) through the performance of others.[12] As we will see shortly, the complexity of this transition is exacerbated by the grounding roots most physicians have as independent and individualistic doers.[13]

The dynamic and daunting nature of this transition cannot be overstated. Consider some of the leadership research that has addressed this theme. In her pioneering research, Harvard professor Linda Hill has vividly described the key transitions that are faced by new, first-time managers.[14] Among her central themes is the difficult transition from "doer" to "leader." Here, Hill argued that this transition represented a profound psychological adjustment that required unlearning deeply held attitudes and habits that had been developed and engaged over years as individual performers.[15] In a similar vein, we have written about the career transitions of emerging leaders in their 20s and 30s who encounter the problematic initial transition from respected individual performer to leader.[16]

The complexity of this transition is highlighted by some dramatic evidence. For example, the Corporate Leadership Council conducted a six-year study of more than 20,000 high-potential "stars," drawn from more than 100 companies throughout the world.[17] The researchers found that nearly 40 percent of these promising, talented up-and-comers failed as leaders. The study yielded a startling outcome — more than 70 percent of these presumed stars simply did not possess the critical attributes, skills and perspectives needed to address the daunting and unfamiliar challenges of contemporary leadership. In short, while these men and women had been outstanding individual performers, application of their skill sets was insufficient for success in leadership roles. Closely paralleling these findings, a report from Right Management found that about 30 percent of new managers failed in their new jobs where true leadership began to replace reliance on individual initiative.[18]

Consider another study, this time from the high-tech world of Google. Recently, Google, concerned about the problematic nature of its engineers moving into management, dug through volumes of performance reviews and feedback surveys, hoping to glean difference-making insights. The single strongest pitfall involved transitioning from outstanding individual performer to being the leader of a team.[19] The theme continues. Drawing from decades of research, the Center for Creative Leadership found that new managers often struggle and fail because they focus too much on their own abilities and neglect the people they are attempting to lead.[20]

While contexts differ, applications for physician leaders have been noted. For example, in an excellent study, Michael Guthrie described physicians as "doers," experts who place strong value on their autonomy.[21] Moreover, physicians may face additional, somewhat idiosyncratic complications. Experts have suggested that physician leaders face "unique obstacles" in leader roles precisely because of the "professional selection, socialization and training" they have received.[22] In short, physicians are encouraged to develop a strong sense of individuality, autonomy and independence.[23] Part of the physician's doer orientation is built into the very structure of the traditional medical setting, where decisions are made by the individual physician.[24]

One could readily argue that "medicine selects and encourages those capable of individual accomplishment above teamwork. ..."[25] This orientation or mindset, honed and reinforced, cannot and will not be discarded simply because one moves from the examining room to the boardroom. Further, as we noted earlier, physician leaders engage in mixed or blended roles. Engaged as both practicing physicians and facilitative leaders, physicians have to address the demands of both contexts.

All of this underscores the critical nature of the physician's leadership transition. As Ruth Collins-Nakai notes, "Leadership necessarily involves stepping away from the individual physician-patient relationship and examining problems at a systems level, requiring the ability to view issues broadly and systematically."[26]

And there is much more, as we will explore in subsequent chapters. As physician leaders, you must learn to engage others. You will frame visions of future action, but you must allow others to carry them out. You must delegate — a process easier said than done for successful doers. You must coach others and help them grow in both competence and confidence. You must grasp that the truly troubling questions are generally beyond any single person's range of comprehension. You must become comfortable with collective discussions and decision-making — processes that can feel painfully slow and cumbersome.

The Transition from Technical Skills to Interpersonal Skills

Recently, a nonclinical health care administrator shared his frustration in working on a strategic initiative team with a renowned senior surgeon:

"OK, we get it. He is brilliant. He literally wrote the book in his area. But I cringe every time he speaks. Within minutes, he can alienate everybody in the room. We're not idiots, and he has no finesse."

Simplistically yet clearly, the behavioral approach that played so well for the surgeon in the surgical setting was largely ineffective for strategy discussions among presumed peers.

Physicians do not abandon their well-honed technical and specialty skills as they move to leader roles. Indeed, the blended nature of clinical and leadership activities counters any such inclination. However, considerable evidence covering more than 50 years of study underscores that effective leadership requires an additional set of skills that may be underdeveloped and underused. To be effective, physician leaders need systematic training to develop and enhance a new set of skills and competencies, the bulk of which can broadly be classified as interpersonal. Let's consider a few findings.

We have long recognized that technical or focused specialty skills become "relatively" less important as one advances in leadership. This does not mean, especially in a physician context, that technical skills are unimportant. Rather, additional skills — such as conceptual skills, complex problem-solving skills and social judgment skills — rise in importance.[27] While the ability to work with people is key at all levels, the background, needs and expectations of those with whom the physician interacts shift, often requiring a refining of interpersonal and behavioral approaches.[28]

A study of 5,400 new leaders seems particularly pertinent for our physician audience. In this study, researchers distinguished between characteristics of "struggling" and "thriving" leaders. Struggling leaders seemed to get bogged down in details and minutiae; reacted negatively to criticism that addressed areas of weakness; responded in ways that intimidated others; jumped to conclusions and solutions without involving others, and micromanaged others' work.[29]

On the other hand, thriving leaders were able to build relationships, demonstrated empathy and interpersonal sensitivity, gained buy-in from others, and brought people together to work and succeed as a team. In fact, three themes — providing clear expectations, building commitment to a common cause and building rapport and relationships — seemed to be competencies that helped thriving leaders produce impressive results.

Studies have emphasized the importance of these key but hard-to-engage characteristics. For example, a detailed study of nearly 200 successful executives identified the handling of difficult relationships and nuanced political situations, and one's temperament and self-awareness (including acknowledging weaknesses) as being critical to long-term executive success.[30] In another highly regarded investigation, renowned Harvard professor John Kotter emphasized that the three critical functions of leaders are setting the direction, aligning the people and motivating and inspiring.[31]

These broad studies are augmented by additional studies that have focused on the critical skills and competencies needed for effective physician leadership. These include engaging in deep listening and respectful communication; generating persuasive arguments and creating influence and buy-in; demonstrating conflict resolution and negotiation; applying emotional and social intelligence; understanding teamwork and team building; understanding and working effectively in politicized contexts; providing vision; motivating others and leading transformational change.[32]

Let's consider one last study. Drawing from interviews with 25 faculty physicians at the Cleveland Clinic, researchers found four recurring themes that were seen as requisite for those aspiring to leadership positions. These were knowledge — including practical position-related knowledge of finance and budgets, as well as field-related expertise; people skills — including dimensions of emotional intelligence; vision, and organizational orientation

— including understanding the history and operating structure of the organization and a commitment to work for the good of the organization. The people-oriented theme was the most frequently noted.[33]

At this point, three impressions should be considered. First, in spite of the evidence, some physicians have difficulty recognizing the importance of and need for what they refer to as "soft" skills (a phrase that rankles those of us who focus on the intricacies of interpersonal behavior). One of the first tasks we face in working with and coaching physician leaders is gaining an understanding and acceptance that interpersonal skills are profoundly important.

Second, we do not assume that physicians are devoid of key interpersonal skills. Rather, these skills have most likely been underdeveloped.

Third, key interpersonal and behavioral skills and activities can be developed and sharpened. This is the focus of our work together throughout this book.

We are fond of a loosely conceived term that we call "interpersonal finesse." As a physician leader interacting with others, your points may need to be made carefully with an awareness of the full range of points of view and corresponding egos. Manner and tone become important, underscoring the maxim that "it's not what you say but the way you say it." Political exchanges become a requirement as you move from one answer to a blended, negotiated approach that is necessary to enhance the probability of acceptance and execution. Conceding on minor points to build social credit for more important issues is critical.

Physicians may verbalize the value of interpersonal skills. However, the true impact and underlying importance of these skills becomes sharper as one experiences new decision-making contexts. In administrative contexts, a plethora of outcomes are in the mix. These include such touchy realities as cost management, quality assurances, complex analytics and metrics (that are presumed to lead to better patient care) and patient-centered models. Here, agendas are mixed. Vested interests are always at play.

Within the realm of these complexities, shared decision-making is expected. Pushing hard and demanding a victory may win the day but inhibit one's potential to build support needed for tomorrow's issues. Except in rare cases, one who fumbles in the interpersonal arena will have a hard time being effective and satisfied in the leadership realm.

The Transition from Change Reactor to Change Leader

Change defines the world of contemporary health care. Physicians, as specialists within a maze of complexity and volatility, live with both awareness of and sensitivity to the need to adjust, innovate, anticipate and realign. Yet these are largely reactor roles. There is nothing pejorative or diminishing about such a claim. And the assumption certainly recognizes that physicians are progressive, forward-thinking people. Rather, it is a reflection of a unique and valued perspective within a turbulent system. Technical specialists, regardless of their talents, are always looking for ways to do their work (medical care) and meet the needs of their clientele (patients) with greater diligence and success. These are fundamentally pursuits to maximize success within a given system.

Leadership is different. Here, one is asked to be a change leader rather than a change reactor. Here, one is asked to reinvent, initiate and lead others to accept and engage in a new world of expanded visions. It is not our intent — or our expertise — to enter in the dynamics of progressive health care debates yet we recognize that this is precisely what is expected of physician leaders.

We are also aware of certain harsh realities. Research tells us that most change initiatives started each year fail, and even more daunting, between 80 and 90 percent of new initiatives fail to meet intended goals and fall short of being seen as successes.[34] Perhaps most bothersome is a phenomenon known as "initiative decay," where new initiatives fail to take hold and are abandoned before they gain traction.[35]

Although we will explore the dynamics of change leadership much more fully in a later chapter, certain themes are relevant to our discussion at this point. Some of the unfortunate failures noted above no doubt are a product of poorly envisioned and weakly crafted change initiatives. Even the most talented leaders can misread and misfire in a turbulent environment. Yet evidence suggests that this generally is not the case. Rather, most failures are due to poorly conceived patterns of execution — designs that pay too little attention to the complex personal, emotional and behavioral dynamics that can thwart even the grandest strategy.[36]

The physician leader is expected to make a critical impact in this expanded arena of change. This potential exists precisely because physicians possess unique perspectives that non-clinicians do not. You bring to the strategy table an awareness of the complexities that change has on the medical practice. You understand patient needs, and you have insight, authenticity and credibility to help build acceptance among other clinicians who are charged with "making it happen." There is an important caveat here. Namely, these possibilities for positive change occur only when physician leaders like you have appropriate behavioral sensitivities to deal with resistance and activate others.

A Transition in Identity

There is a fourth and final transition that is deeply personal. Whether we use the terms inner reorientation, self-definition or transition in mindset, the move from clinician to a blended model of physician leadership involves some degree of personal reorientation of self-identity. We will tip, ever so broadly, into some focused thinking on the nature of identity and its applications for physician leaders.

Strong conceptual foundations, drawn from a variety of disciplinary perspectives, have yielded several theoretical views of identity. These models — such as social identity theory, self-categorization theory and collective identity — have helped us gain a deeper understanding of how one's identity is comprised and organized.[37] Within these theories, terms such as "identity salience," "psychological centrality" and identity "importance" help clarify how membership in a specific group contributes to our overall sense of self.[38]

After years of study, training and practice, the physician identity is quite ingrained. Further, one's physician identity transcends immediate work situations and touches the physician's "everyday ongoing social relationships" — a factor known as "social embeddedness."[39] All of this leads to a conclusion that each of you no doubt intuits: The physician identity is paramount, and it carries significant degrees of personal pride, interpersonal prestige and social status. The depth and significance of one's physician identity can hardly be overstated.

Let's briefly consider another, related view. Researchers have provided evidence that most people experience one of three distinct relationships with their work: Work is seen as a "job," work is seen as a "career," or work is seen as a "calling."[40] People who have "jobs" view their work in purely instrumental terms, and work is a means for attaining resources that will enable them to secure enjoyment outside of the job. In contrast, people who view their work as a "career" have a "deeper personal investment in their work and mark their achievements not only through monetary gain, but [also] through advancement within the organizational structure" … leading to "higher social standing, increased power … and higher self-esteem."[41]

The view of work as a "calling" is markedly different and distinct. Here, people find that work is integral to and largely inseparable from who they are and the life they live. The primary reason for work is neither financial advantage nor career advancement. Instead, one works for the experiences of personal fulfillment and meaning.

Additionally, those who view their work as a calling see work not only as enhancing their lives but as contributing to some noble cause. Not surprisingly, people who see their work as a calling experience their work as highly rewarding, tend to be dedicated workers, and consequently are likely to be quite successful in their work.[42]

While admittedly generalized, our work suggests that physicians engage their clinical work as a calling, and the "noble cause" commentary clearly resonates. Experts concur, noting that a physician's sense of personal meaning and significance (intrinsic value) is drawn from the doctor/patient relationship.[43] We hear anecdotal affirmations of this on a regular basis. "Despite all that's going on in health care, I love my patients — they're what counts." Or, "This (the patient relationship) is why I got into medicine in the first place." Compounding this orientation is the belief among many doctors that few people care about the patient the way they do.[44]

There is a final piece to the identity considerations. Physicians tend to have strong professional orientations and commitments that involve both identity and loyalty. Generally, this translates into being more concerned with maintaining the standards and expectations of the profession than those of any particular employing organization. Further, when conflicting expectations arise, the presumed demands of the profession predominate.

The setup is clear. We have already established that physician leaders engage in blended roles — spending part of their time as clinicians and part as leaders. As such, some degree of reshaping of identity occurs, and the process can be conflictual. At times, physicians fight to maintain their physician identity, even while serving in leader roles. While reasonable and natural, this can be restrictive. As such, it is critical to embrace your leader identity and allow both centers of significance to flourish.

William Bridges' groundbreaking book *Transitions: Making Sense of*

Life Changes offers important and thoughtful insights that seem particularly relevant for our discussion.[45] Bridges draws a key distinction between change and transition. In short, he argues that while change is situational (i.e., moving from one job to another), transition is psychological — that is deeply personal and emotional. Accordingly, transition involves an "inner reorientation" and "self-redefinition." Critically, Bridges argues that change is doomed without transition, a point that subsequent work has supported and reinforced.[46]

The connections here are important, and they are especially relevant for physician leaders. Further, they are a key to why we have conceptualized the physician-to-physician leader change as a transition. Transitions succeed only when we realize that there will have to be new beginnings. These beginnings typically involve the development of new skills, taking a new and more encompassing look at things and allowing our worldview to be redefined, reshaped and expanded. Tossed into the fray, these new beginnings become trickier and far more complicated than expected when we observe rather than occupy the leader's chair.

Strengths and Vulnerabilities

We conclude this chapter on a cautionary note by suggesting that some of the characteristics and tendencies that have facilitated success in your clinical role may, if overplayed, be detrimental in leadership roles. The effort here is not to minimize the formidable nature of these strengths. Rather, the purpose is to suggest that a keen awareness of and perhaps tempering may be needed in the leadership context. We often hear two rejoinders to this call: "I can't change who I am," and, "This is who I am, deal with it." However, we all have the capacity to engage situations differently, displaying key aspects of emotional intelligence and impulse control — topics we will explore fully in later chapters.

Bob Kaplan and Rob Kaiser, in their book *Fear Your Strengths*, provide an in-depth and fascinating perspective on what most of us recognize in others but may fail to see in ourselves. Drawing from extensive assessments of senior executives, the authors concluded that when leaders overemphasized certain key strengths, their overall leadership effectiveness was compromised.[47]

An example may be helpful. Recently, we worked with the leadership team of a midsized health care practice that had hired a new leader to offer stronger financial skills and provide deeper levels of business acumen to the operations. Within his first six months, the leader met and exceeded most performance expectations. Armed with strong financial metrics, he refocused the organization's thinking, decision-making and evaluative criteria. Clear metrics, enhanced measurement and timely adjustments were the watchwords of a new cultural orientation.

As you might expect, strict adherence to metrics was perceived by many in the practice as becoming so dominant that individuality, attention to the personal dimensions of employees and patients, and interpersonal communication were secondary considerations, if they were considered at all. Seeing some evidence of these impressions at play, the leader's immediate response was to turn to what he knew best and where he was most comfortable. He engaged in extended, unilateral assessments of key performance outcomes, reducing individuals and units to key performance indicators.

Predictably, this approach produced further alienation within the practice. It is easy to say that he overplayed his strengths and excluded key insights on change leadership. Yet playing to his strengths and focusing on where he excelled was natural.

We all have this tendency to play to our areas of strength, and both research and practical perspective have shown the efficacy of this approach. In fact, an entire philosophical view of leadership has focused on identifying, maximizing and capitalizing on strengths rather than engaging in burdensome (and often ineffective) efforts to ameliorate our shortcomings.[48]

Caution, however, is important. Certain shortcomings should be ameliorated as they can destroy interpersonal effectiveness and derail a leader's success.[49] Not surprisingly, some of these potential shortcomings are offshoots of areas of strength and competency.[50]

Consider the following. The Center for Creative Leadership has conducted extensive research on why leaders fail or derail.[51] Seven characteristics are common: an abrasive, intimidating style; coldness and arrogance; untrustworthiness; self-centeredness and overly political behaviors; poor communication; poor performance, and inability to delegate.[52] In many cases, the negativity of these characteristics is exacerbated by one's poor evaluations of the situational dynamics (where it takes place and who is present), caustic conversational tone and a general lack of interpersonal finesse.

Armed with this perspective, let's look at a few physician strengths and the shadow side of these strengths. It's important to repeat our earlier caveat — we are drawing generalized themes that have evidential basis, but they will not be applicable across all people and contexts.

Intelligence and Action-Orientation

To state the obvious, physicians are intelligent and well-educated. It is likely that as you sit around the table with other health care administrators, your broad intellectual firepower will exceed that of most others in the room. There is no need for self-deprecating denials. It's more important to acknowledge this scenario and move to understand the opportunities and complexities that come with this background.

We often ask our physician audiences a research question. What would you hypothesize is the relationship between intelligence and leader effectiveness? Although intelligence is a complex construct, research has consistently shown a positive relationship between intelligence and leader effectiveness, especially when parceled and refined into what is referred to as analytic intelligence or general problem-solving ability.[53]

However, there is a bit more to the story. Evidence suggests and many leadership experts believe that the relationship between analytic intelligence and leader effectiveness is actually curvilinear.[54] That is, as one's level of intelligence rises, so does leader effectiveness — up to a point or threshold level. As one's intelligence exceeds this level or moves substantially beyond that of the work team, one actually becomes less effective as a leader.

Thinking this through, multiple explanations emerge as culprits, but the most parsimonious explanation has to do with the difficulty of connecting and communicating with others. There is also some feeling that if leaders possess levels of intelligence that are considerably higher than others on the team, their ideas may simply be too advanced for others to accept. Accordingly, while leaders tend to possess higher intelligence than non-leaders, effectiveness is maintained when the gap is not substantial.[55]

Let's consider a related theme. Physicians, generally, are quick studies. To a large extent, the nature and demands of the clinical setting require one to quickly gather data, draw conclusions and provide answers. In most cases, this capacity has been learned and honed through years of clinical orientation and practice. There are also important leadership advantages here. For example, research indicates that being a quick study can be a key to effective leadership in today's fast-paced environment.[56]

Being an intelligent, quick study leads to another characteristic. Physicians tend to be decisive decision-makers. Basically, decisiveness is conceptualized as the capacity to make decisions (presumably sound decisions) with incomplete information. Again, research evidence indicates that decisiveness is a key for leader success, particularly in volatile, competitive environments such as those encountered in health care.[57] Further, a lack of appropriate decisiveness is often revealed as a factor undermining or derailing one's leadership progress. And, not surprisingly, a lack of decisiveness emerges as one of the foremost struggles faced by new and emerging leaders.

Part of the capacity for decisiveness is based on what we term "probability thinking" — an area where physicians excel. Here, rather than striving for complete and undeniably clear evidence before proceeding to action, probability thinking involves tradeoffs, realizing that delays in responding carry important opportunity costs. Acceptable levels of probable outcomes and assurances are weighed against the costs of delaying for additional evidence that may never arrive; and also reduce the possible range of future options through inaction.

Linked with the issues noted here are four physician tendencies that are laudatory. First, physicians tend to have extremely high standards of personal performance excellence. Second, physicians expect others to have high levels of technical expertise and competency in their respective areas. Third, physicians expect performance outcomes of the highest level. Fourth, physicians, generally, have little tolerance for those who fall short in meeting competency and performance expectations.

The Shadow Side of Intelligence and Action-Orientation

Drawing from the points noted above, there can be a shadow side that manifests in a leadership context where one must work with and through others who hold various positions of authority and represent diverse disciplines. Physicians are at times perceived as having impatience toward others. We hear the comments from our physician audiences. "We're wasting time."

"We are discussing the obvious." "Come on, make a decision already."

Our consulting and research across broad groups of technical experts who move into positions of leadership suggest that impatience is a common theme. It occurs among highly trained engineers assuming leader roles. It is encountered among information technology experts moving into new leadership positions. And it occurs in many cases among physician leaders who assume the mantle of leadership.

Candid realism is helpful here. As a leader, you will now be drawn into projects, meetings and sessions with talented people from a range of backgrounds. It is likely that some of these people simply will not grasp and assess data and reach conclusions as readily as you. Rather than lamenting the obvious, it is more prudent to accept this reality of and practice behaviors to address the situation.

While this theme will reoccur at times through this book, certain points must be addressed up front. First, impatience is rarely masked without careful, dedicated and focused action. Impatience can emerge from blunt and caustic (albeit honest and correct) commentary during meetings. Or, even more common, impatience flashes forward through clear nonverbal signals.

Those on the receiving end are generally accomplished and proud organizational members. As such, actions of impatience are experienced as being disrespectful and diminishing — undercutting one's need for personal significance. Understandably, people recoil at this, draw quick perceptions and target the perpetrator as being arrogant and dismissive. As a result, the spiral of negative interpersonal currency is spinning.

Physician leaders can also be seen as inflexible. In part, drawing from training and experience, doctors can appear intransigent once their minds are made up. We recall the honest words of a talented surgeon who opined, "This is my patient. I know what needs to be done. I will listen, but I know what needs to be done." The surgeon found that while this perspective was relatively effective in a clinical setting, it created animosity when working with other organizational leaders on team-oriented projects. His approach fostered natural barriers, defensiveness and team tension.

Additionally, physicians may be perfectionists who find that others consistently fall short of their expectations. The response here is not to lower expectations. Rather, selectivity, clarity and sensitivity are needed. In simplest terms, selectivity suggests that every issue need not be taken to the mat

— every point of difference need not be a battle. Picking the critical issues that cannot be compromised or neglected and differentiating these from the broader range of potential issues is an important initial step. Being very clear — crystal clear — regarding needed expectations around these issues is the next step. Third, and most critical, steps one and two must progress with an open, non-dogmatic, inclusive and engaged interpersonal style.

Physicians, drawing from a tendency to grasp issues quickly and move decisively, may have underdeveloped listening skills, especially when working in a cross-disciplinary team. In part, this comes from a history of selective informational listening. Drawing from clinical backgrounds, there can be a tendency to listen for specific pieces of data or evidence that will clarify and solidify assessments and paths of remediation. Listening for the understory, which is often masked and indirectly presented, is a different skill. Further, the understory is often a manifestation of unmet needs that percolate at a deep and emotional level. Skills in this critical area will be addressed in a later chapter.

Physicians are at times accused of preferring action over behavioral sensitivity. This preference is no doubt the product of one's intelligence, quick grasp of complex issues and resulting decisiveness. As noted earlier, all these preferences can be important leader strengths.

Fortunately or unfortunately, as one advances in leadership and decisions become more strategic, incremental decision-making tends to prevail. Incremental decision-making is not indecisiveness. Rather, it is the realization that decisions have broad consequence and impact and, as such, normally progress through stages and levels of involvement in the organization. Of course, such a decision-making approach can be frustrating. Further, there is no doubt that the process unfolds far too slowly in many organizations, especially given the immediate health care quagmire with which we must grapple.

Yet incremental decision-making is based on a belief in checks and balances and garnering acceptance from key constituencies. The logic here suggests that incremental decision-making provides the greatest assurance of correct strategic moves and enhances the likelihood of successful implementation.

High Achievers

Physicians are likely to possess both a high need for achievement and its corollary, a high need to avoid failure.[58] These characteristics have received extensive, broad-ranging research consideration.[59] Three characteristics are common among those who are high on the need for achievement scale.

First, high achievers do not want outcomes left to chance. That is, they want to be sure that outcomes are the result of their efforts rather than those of external factors (luck, fate and especially less competent others).

Second, high achievers tend to set moderately difficult but potentially achievable goals for themselves. In common parlance, these are known as "personal stretch goals." Indeed, the stretch is part of the challenge, excitement and energizing impact of throwing oneself into a task.

The third characteristic is a bit more complicated. High achievers desire direct, concrete and timely feedback regarding the efficacy of their actions and performance. Accordingly, they tend to gravitate toward activities that provide these feedback dimensions. Not surprisingly, one of the frustrations that high achievers encounter in leadership roles comes from the lag between action and feedback. Clear, tangible and immediate feedback appears to be missing, and deferred feedback is more common, especially for longer-range strategic actions.

The need for achievement produces amazing drive and plays a critical role in the physician's inner motivation. However, there is also a shadow side that can be problematic. For example, drawing from a strong need for achievement, physicians are likely to take a hands-on approach to tasks that can minimize the contributions of others on the team.[60] At times, physicians' drive to achieve can be seen by others as the need to win, or even more questionable, to "win at all costs."

The transition to leadership requires an honest assessment of your formidable strengths and how these strengths are expressed in various interpersonal contexts. In many cases, your strengths may need to be displayed judiciously, often with tempering behaviors.

For example, your drive to achieve may need to be coupled with emotional self-awareness; an ability to "read" how behaviors are coming across to others; heavy doses of affirmations and earned praise directed toward others; and clearly demonstrated respect for others. Your decisiveness may need an early check, augmented by open-ended questions that involve others. Your action orientation may need to be "paced down" so others can accept ideas and feel a sense of personal ownership. These need not be diminishing behaviors. Rather, the hope and promise is that your strengths gain deeper credibility within a broader context — the context of leadership.

Concluding Thoughts

Self-assured and in his early 40s, Kendell Lancaster is an excellent physician with a fierce dedication to his patients. Administrators within his organization felt that his impassioned and somewhat idealistic views were exactly what was needed as a new specialty center was being considered. Six months later, these same non-clinical leaders blanched at their naïve and foolish decision. Lancaster proved to be "cantankerous, bullheaded and abrasive." Conclusions were clear. "He can't lead, and he can't work with others."

Cautiously agreeing to work with Lancaster, we had no idea what to expect. We found him to be a strong-willed perfectionist punctuated by a sense of intellectual assurance. We also liked him, concluding that his combination of competence, confidence and procedural certainty was exactly what we wanted from a doctor.

Yet he could be tough to engage. He questioned nearly everything — a quality that no doubt translated as over-opinionated and argumentative. He was bluntly insensitive, issuing matter-of-fact pronouncements as unassailable bursts of wisdom. He rarely offered praise for "just doing what's expected." And he had a bothersome tendency of processing input but never commenting on others' ideas and perspectives — a tendency that others saw as dismissive.

Moving into a leadership position, Lancaster had not adjusted. He had not recognized the impact of a different organizational context. He had not transitioned. His story has helped frame this chapter. In the words of executive coach and author Marshall Goldsmith, "What got you here won't get you there."[61] Leadership is a different world. Let's get started.

....

1.   Kornacki, M.J. & Silversin, J. (2012). *Leading Physicians through Change: How to Achieve and Sustain Results.* (2nd edition). Tampa, FL: American College of Physician Executives.

2.   Guthrie, M.B. (1999). Challenges in developing physician leadership and management. *Frontiers of Health Services Management,* 15(4), 3-26.

3.   Hicks, R. & McCracken, J. (2014). The motivational profile of an effective physician leader. *Physician Executive,* 40 (3), 102-105.

4.   Stoller, J.K. (2008). Developing physician-leaders: Key competencies and available programs. *The Journal of Health Administration Education,* Fall, 307-328.

5.   Beehr, T.A.; Nair, V.N.; Gudanowski, D.M.; & Such, M. (2004). Perceptions of reasons for promotion of self and others. *Human Relations,* 57(4), 413-438.

6.   Ibarra, H.; Snook, S.; & Ramo, L.G. (2010). Identity-based leadership development. In N. Nohria & R. Khurana (Eds.). *Handbook of leadership theory and practice,* Boston: Harvard Business Press, p. 666.

7. Barnhart, G. & O'Brien, M. (2008). Overcoming physician leadership limbo. *Healthcare Executive,* 28(1), 88, 90.

8. Kabir, C.; Potty, A.; & Sharma, R. (2008). Current opportunities for the development of leadership skills in doctors. *The International Journal of Clinical Leadership,* 16, 115-119. Dowton, S.B. (2004). Leadership in medicine: Where are the leaders? *Medical Journal of Australia,* 181, 652-654.

9. Clark, J.; Spurgeon, P.; & Hamilton, P. (2008). Medical professionalism: Leadership complexity — an essential ingredient. *The International Journal of Clinical Leadership,* 16, 2-9.10.

11. Magill, M.K. (1998). Becoming an effective physician leader. *Family Practice Management,* 6, 35-37.12.

13. Fairchild, D.G.; Benjamin, E.M.; Gifford, D.R.; & Huot, S.J. (2004). Physician leadership: Enhancing the career development of academic physician administrators and leaders. *Academic Medicine,* 79(3), 214-218, p. 214.

14. Stoner, C.R., & Stoner, J.S. (2013). *Building Leaders: Paving the Path for Emerging Leaders.* New York: Routledge.

15. Sangvai, D.; Lyn, M.; & Michener, L. (2008). Defining high-performance teams and physician leadership. *The Physician Executive,* March-April, 44-51.

16. Hill, L.A. (2003). *Becoming a Manager: How New Managers Master the Challenges of Leadership.* Boston: Harvard Business School Press.

17. Ibid.

18. Stoner & Stoner, 2013.

19. Martin, J. & Schmidt, C. (2010). How to keep your top talent. *Harvard Business Review,* 88(5), 54-61.

20. Williams, R. (2010, May 2). CEO failures: How on-boarding can help [Blog]. Received from www.psychologytoday.com/blog/wired-success/201005/ceo-failures-how-onboarding-can-help.

21. Harrison, A.J. (2011). *Google's management rules.* Retrieved from http://andrewjohnharrison.com/.

22. Gentry, W.A. It's not about me. It's about me & you. How being dumped can help first-time managers. Center for Creative Leadership White Paper. Greensboro, NC: Center for Creative Leadership.

23. Guthrie, 1999.

24. Ibid., p. 5.

25. Sangvai, et al., 2008.

26. Snell, A.J.; Briscoe, D.; & Dickson, G. (2011). From the inside out: The engagement of physicians as leaders in health care settings. *Qualitative Health Research,* 21(7), 952-967.

27. Ibid., p. 47.

28. Collins-Nakai, R. (2006). Leadership in medicine. *McGill Journal of Medicine,* 9, 68-73, p. 68.

29. Katz, R.L. (1955). The skills of an effective administrator, *Harvard Business Review,* 33(1), 33-42. Mumford, M.D.; Zacarro, S.J.; Harding, F.D.; Jacobs, T.O.; & Fleishman, E.A. (2000). Leadership skills for a changing world: Solving complex social problems. *Leadership Quarterly,* 11(1), 11-35.

30. Mumford, M.D.; Zacarro, S.J.; Harding, F.D.; Jacobs, T.O.; & Fleishman, E.A. (2000). Leadership skills for a changing world: Solving complex social problems. *Leadership Quarterly,* 11(1), 11-35.

31. Van Buren, M. & Safferstone, T. (2009). The quick wins paradox. *Harvard Business Review,* 87(1), 54-61.

32. McCall, M.W.; Lombardo, M.M.; & Morrison, A.M. (1988). *The Lessons of Experience: How Successful Executives Develop on the Job.* Lexington, MA: Lexington Books.

33. Kotter, J.P. (2001). What leaders really do. *Harvard Business Review,* 79(11), 85-96.

34. Ciampa, E.J.; Hunt, A.A.; Arneson, K.O.; Mordes, D.A.; Oldham, W.M.; Vin Woo, K.; Owens, D.A.; Cannon, M.D.; & Dermody, T.S. (2011). A workshop for MD/PhD students. *Medical Education Online,* 16: 7075 – DOI: 10.3402/meo.v1610.7075. Mckenna, M.K.; Gartland, M.P.; & Pugno, P.A. (2004). Development of physician leadership competencies: Perceptions of physician leaders, physician educators, and medical students. *Journal of Health Administration Education,* 21, 343-354. Santric Milicevic, M.M.; Bjegovic-Mikanovic, V.M.; Terzic-Supic, Z.J.; & Vasic, V. (2011). *European Journal of Public Health,* 21, 247-253. Taylor, C.A.; Taylor, J.C.; & Soller, J.K. (2008). Exploring physician competencies in established and aspiring physician leaders: An interview-based study. *Journal of General Internal Medicine,* 23(6), 748-754.35.

36. Taylor, Taylor, & Stoller, 2008.

37. Beer, M. & Nohria, N. (2000). Cracking the code of change. *Harvard Business Review,* 78(3), 133-141. IBM Business Consulting Services. (2004). *Your Turn: The Global CEO Study of 2004.* Retrieved from http://www-05.ibm.com/no/news/publications/IBI. Karp, T. & Helgo, T.I.T. (2009). Reality revisited: Leading people in chaotic change. *Journal of Management Development,* 28(2), 81-93.38.

39. Doyle, M.; Claydon, T.; & Buchanan, D. (2000). Mixed results, lousy process: Contrasts and contradictions in the management experience of change. *British Journal of Management,* 11, 59-80.

40. Heath & Heath. (2010). Kotter, J.P. & Cohen, D.S. (2002). *The Heart of Change: Real-Life Stories of How People Change Their Organizations.* Boston: Harvard Business School Publishing. Labianca, et al. (2000).

41. Brubaker, R. & Cooper, F. (2000). Beyond "identity." *Theory and Society,* 29,1-47. Stryker, S. (1980). *Sybolic Interactionism.* Menlo Park, CA: Benjamin/Cummings. Tajfel, H. (1982). *Social Identity and Intergroup Relations.* Cambridge, UK: Cambridge University Press.

42. Ashmore, R.D.; Deaux, K.; & McLaughlin-Volpe, T. (2004). An organizing framework for collective identity: Articulation and significance of multidimensionality. *Psychological Bulletin,* 130, 80-114. Rosenberg, M. (1979). *Conceiving the Self.* New York: Basic Books.

43. Ashmore, *et al.*

44. Wrzesniewski, A.; McCauley, C.; Rozin, P.; & Schwartz, B. (1997). Jobs, careers, and callings: People's relations to their work. *Journal of Research in Personality,* 31(1), 21-33.

45. Ibid., p.22.

46. Achor, S. (2010). *The Happiness Advantage: The Seven Principles of Positive Psychology That Fuel Success and Performance at Work.* New York: Crown Business.

47. Ellis, B.M.; Rutter, P.; Greaves, F.; Noble, D.; Lemer, B. (2011). New models of clinical leadership: The chief medical officer clinical advisor scheme. *The International Journal of Clinical Leadership,* 17, 1-6.

48. Guthrie, B. (1999). Challenges in developing physician leadership and management. *Frontiers of Health Services Management,* 15(4), 3-26.

49. Bridges, W. (2004). *Transitions: Making Sense of Life's Changes.* (2nd ed.). Cambridge, MA: First Da Capo Press.

50. Heath, C. & Heath, D. (2010). *Switch: How to Change When Change Is Hard.* New York: Broadway Books. Kotter, J. (1996). *Leading Change.* Boston: Harvard Business School Press. Labianco, G.; Gray, B.; & Brass, D.J. (2000). A grounded model of organizational schema change during empowerment. *Organization Science,* 11, 235-257.51.

52. Kaplan, R.E. & Kaiser, R.B. (2013). *Fear Your Strengths: What You Are Best at Could Be Your Biggest Problem.* San Francisco, CA: Berrett-Koehler.

53. Buckingham, M. & Clifton, D.O. (2001). *Now Discover Your Strengths.* New York: Simon & Schuster.

54. Leslie, J.B. (2003). *Leadership and Skills of Emotional Intelligence.* Greensboro, NC: The Center for Creative Leadership.

55. Hogan, J.; Hogan, R.; & Kaiser, R.B. (2010). Management derailment. In S. Zedeck (ed.). *American Psychological Association Handbook of Industrial and Organizational Psychology,* vol.3, Washington, D.C.: American Psychological Association, pp. 555-575.

56. McCall, M.W. & Lombardo, M.M. (1983). Off the track: Why and how successful executives get derailed. Technical Report No. 21. Greensboro, NC: The Center for Creative Leadership.

57. Nahavandi, A. (2012). *The Art and Science of Leadership.* Upper Saddle River, NJ: Prentice Hall, p. 128.

58. Sternberg, R.J. (1997). The concept of intelligence: Its role in lifelong learning and success. *American Psychologist,* 52(10), 1030-1037.

59. Stogdill, R.M. (1974). *The Handbook of Leadership.* New York: Free Press.60.

61. Northouse, P.G. *Leadership: Theory and Practice.* (5h ed.). Thousand Oaks, CA: Sage.62.

63. Patterson, T.E.; Champion, H.; Browning, H.; Torain, D.; Harrison, C.; Gurvis, J.; Fleenor, J.; & Campbell, M. (2011). Addressing the leadership gap in healthcare: What's needed when it comes to leader talent. Center for Creative Leadership White Paper. Greensboro, NC: The Center for Creative Leadership.

64. Ibid.

65. Hicks, R. & McCracken, J. (2014). The motivational profile of an effective physician leader. *Physician Executive,* 40(3), 102-105.

66. Atkinson, J.S. & Feather, N.T. (1966). *A Theory of Achievement Motivation.* New York: John Wiley & Sons. McClelland, D.C. (1967). *The Achieving Society.* New York: Free Press. McClelland, D.C. (1976). *The Achievement Motive.* New York: Irvington.

67. Hicks & McCracken, 2014.

68. Goldsmith, M. & Reiter, M. (2007). *What Got You Here Won't Get You There.* New York: Hyperion.

3

Tone: The Significance
of the Interpersonal Factor

....

IN THE PREVIOUS CHAPTER, WE DISCUSSED THE COMPLEX NATURE
of the transition from clinician to physician leader. As we differentiated
successful and thriving leaders from those whose effectiveness was more
limited, the significance of interpersonal sensitivity and behavioral skills and
competencies were highlighted. This chapter extends these themes as we delve
deeply into the dynamics of the interpersonal factor.

We begin by emphasizing the value of interpersonal and relational factors
at work. Here, we must be careful. It is relatively easy to say we value the human
factor at work. In fact, one would be naïve to express the contrary, especially
when the socially appropriate organizational response is so obvious. Yet there
is a difference between saying it, believing it and enacting it. Believing in the
value of interpersonal sensitivity is a deeply personal conviction that reveals
one's underlying attitudes and core values. Enacting — that tell-tale series of
behaviors — takes time, thoughtful consideration and repetition.

By virtue of your credibility and status, you are likely to set the interpersonal tone of your meetings and exchanges. Your tone permeates and
dramatically affects every person and every context you touch. Your tone
affects the practice and organization, playing a dramatic role in defining and
framing the culture that emerges and is experienced by others. Nurses, staff,
administrators, other physicians and even patients are often keenly affected
by your idiosyncratic tone.

When you rush into a meeting, late and harried, move straight to the
facts, and split your attention between the meeting and the iPhone in your
hand, you are setting a tone. At best, the messages and foundational tone

are mixed. At worst, the tone is that you have more important and pressing needs and the current exchanges are a distraction. Those in attendance are likely to feel diminished and disrespected. You can argue that these are not your intentions. You can argue that your world is frazzled and that time is your most precious resource. All of this may be true. But you are still setting a tone that affects everything that follows.

In some cases, clinicians (similar to other highly skilled professionals) approach relational themes with cynicism, unconvinced and unwilling to embrace the value of the interpersonal factor at work. Here, we uncover statements such as "They hired me for my skills, not my personality," and, "If I'm good enough, I shouldn't have to worry about all these interpersonal niceties." These comments reveal a common mindset — "talent trumps likability." As one might expect, leaders rarely assert these views publicly. In fact, they offer a rather sanitized, socially appropriate version espousing the values of teamwork, cooperation and empathy. Despite the rhetoric, deeply ingrained assumptions remain, often reinforced through years of direct experience.

As we will explore in this chapter, these dismissive and minimizing assumptions are broadly inconsistent with research evidence and accepted best practices. Increasingly, research has helped us understand that the leader's emotional tone affects important organizational outcomes.

Leadership and Interpersonal Tone

At its core, all leadership is a relational activity. Successful leaders get this, and struggling leaders do not.

With our competitive survival at stake, we expect a lot from our leaders. Contemporary leaders must foster powerful and centering visions. They must create winning strategies that navigate the shifting nuances of patient needs, demographic realignments, competitive complexities and political and economic realities. They must exercise creativity and innovate, and they must do so in a world of uncertainty and risk. We want and need leaders who are careful purveyors of the future. We want and need astute thinkers who are capable of formulating and framing big ideas that will drive us forward. And yet it is not enough.

Even the most brilliant visionaries and most insightful strategists will experience diminished impact until they master relational and interpersonal skills that enable them to connect with, align and inspire the people around them. Daniel Goleman, Richard Boyatzis and Annie McKee have offered a clear and succinct summary, "Even if they do everything else right, if leaders fail in this primal task of driving emotions in the right direction, nothing they do will work as well as it could or should."[1]

Increasingly, research has emphasized the importance of the leader's interpersonal sensitivity — a specific concept that includes such factors as the ability to identify and appreciate the feelings and perceptions of others; the capacity to view employees as unique and idiosyncratic; and the capacity to display a genuine interest in the employee as a person.[2]

Evidence suggests that employees desire and expect such sensitivity from good leaders and express higher levels of satisfaction when working for interpersonally sensitive leaders, as opposed to their less sensitive counterparts.[3] And, since you were probably wondering, meta-analyses have shown a gender differential. In general, women display more interpersonal sensitivity than men.[4]

The interpersonal impact is far-reaching. Consider all the lauded and needed changes with which we are all involved. Strikingly and perhaps surprisingly, the majority of change initiatives introduced each year will either fail or fall so significantly short of expectations that they cannot be viewed as successes.[5] In most cases, these failures are not due to deficiencies in ideas, visions, strategies or plans. Instead, the failures occur because of fumbled execution that underestimates and devalues the intensity of emotional and relational undertones that build into deep pockets of resistance, thus eroding the heart of successful change.[6]

Or, consider another expansive set of research, reporting that leaders who "stumbled" and found their careers "stalled" or "derailed" experienced a common central theme — difficulties with interpersonal relationships.[7] In fact, these problematic leaders displayed tendencies to intimidate others; react negatively to criticism; jump to conclusions (rather than engaging others and gaining support), and micromanage and meddle in the work of others.

All of this leads to a fascinating series of studies that directly touch the physician's world. Like many behaviorists, we initially were introduced to the research of Nalini Ambady as her work was profiled in the book *Blink*.[8] A noted Stanford University psychologist, Ambady and her colleagues conducted studies that greatly expanded our understanding of the nuances of medical malpractice litigation. These studies, covering the past quarter century, have indicated that patient perception of poor quality was a necessary but not primary condition for pursuing legal action against a physician; patients did not sue physicians whom they liked; and patients' decisions to sue or not were largely determined by how they felt they were treated on a personal level — a decision that was critically affected by the interpersonal and communicative connection between the physician and patient.[9]

As with all research findings, varied views of the implications of the reported evidence are likely, and the studies reported by Ambady and her colleagues are no exception. Given this caveat, we are struck by the impact of key behavioral sensitivities and the profound consequences that arise from patients' perceptions of the relationship that emerges (or fails to emerge) with their physician.

Expanding this theme, the impact denoted here transfers to other contexts and people with whom physicians interface. The nature of your interpersonal relationships at work and the way you treat others on a personal basis can be dramatic. Make no mistake, by virtue of your expertise and status, you create impressions that dominate the tone and mood of those around you. We are fond of the practical observation "the leader's mood is contagious."[10]

Let's return to the work of Ambady and her colleagues. Part of their work centered on micro-level factors, including such subtle perceptions as a physician's tone of voice. Here, research found that a tone of voice labeled as "dominant" — crisp, moderately fast, deep and loud — was often perceived by the patient as lacking empathy and true understanding of the patient. In contrast, "concern" (and even "anxiety") in the tone of voice was associated with perceptions of both empathy and genuine regard for the patient. Not surprisingly, "dominance coupled with a lack of anxiety in the voice may imply surgeon indifference and lead a patient to launch a malpractice suit when poor outcomes occur."[11]

These attributional dynamics are fascinating and suggest how feelings of indifference and dismissiveness can be perceived from a factor as basic as one's tone of voice. These studies help underscore the time-honored wisdom that "how a message is conveyed may be as important as what is said."[12]

In the following sections, we consider important behavioral and interpersonal themes that will help define who you are as a leader, and the impact you create. Realistically, you will see connections among them — how consideration and application of one theme affects perceptions regarding other themes. Further, the issues we address are not exhaustive. Instead, they are beginning frames that will be refined as we progress. And, we begin in what may be a surprising direction.

The Case for Justice

At a conference of physician leaders, a penetrating question was posed by one of the participants during the Q&A session. "Of all these behavioral themes you have discussed, which is most important?"

Yes, I sensed the problematic nature of this "which of your children do you like best" inquiry. Yet I also knew that an academically laden description of interactive complexities would not suffice. A response was needed, and I opted for … justice.

The themes of justice, along with those of equity and fairness, have deep theoretical foundations. However, before delving into the research and relevant applications, let's consider three examples.

In 2014, Raymond Burse was called out of retirement to assume the presidency of Kentucky State University. In one of his first acts as president, Burse gave back $90,000 of his annual salary so that the lowest paid employees on the university's staff could receive pay increases.[13]

And consider the actions of Rob Garnett, a midlevel leader for a large not-for-profit professional association. Garnett pushes hard and expects high levels of performance from his four-person team. In most years, his team exceeds its goals, and he earns a nice bonus. Enter justice and fairness. Each year, Garnett calls his team members together, fixes their gaze on the bonus check that sits on his desk, and proceeds to write a personal check to each member for one-fifth (their share) of his bonus.

It's easy to dismiss these examples as largely symbolic. Yet the messages that are sent regarding equity and a prevailing sense of justice have pervasive and well-established motivational effects.[14]

Now, consider the obverse, a sad example from the annals of organizational history. Some years ago, plagued by competitive woes that drained the bottom line, General Motors CEO Roger Smith lobbied United Auto Workers president Douglas Fraser for critical union concessions — essentially unprecedented "givebacks" — during tricky contract negotiations. Aware of the competitive plight the company faced, the union membership agreed to accept previously unheard of concessions — all in the name of helping the company survive. On the heels of this "victory," the company's board of directors voted GM's top leaders massive salary increases. Imagine the impact of such unfairness and injustice!

Indeed, perceptions of justice have powerful organizational implications. For example, studies using meta-analysis have reported that organizational justice is a strong predictor of job satisfaction, work commitment, trust and turnover intentions (the desire to leave the job).[15] Further, research has revealed that these relationships hold in both North American and East Asian work contexts (although the effects were stronger in North America than East Asia).[16]

Beyond these factors, behavioral subtleties are also at play. Perceptions of justice and fairness contribute to employees' feelings of self-worth, self-esteem and personal significance. Researchers note that "fair procedures and distribution of rewards communicate symbolic messages that individuals are valued members of a group, thus enhancing their self-esteem and fostering positive relationships with others in the group."[17] And, critically, we recognize that work performance is positively impacted by perceptions of justice.[18]

The case for justice has deep roots. We can trace the academic foundations of organizational justice back to the mid 1960s. The initial focus was on the construct of distributive justice. Distributive justice is seen as "the perceived fairness of the outcomes one receives from a social exchange or interaction."[19] This determination is drawn from one's views of whether the outcomes received are seen as fair or equitable. Drawing from Stacey Adams' pioneering work, we understand that people are likely to judge fairness or equity by evaluating their perceived contributions relative to the outcomes they receive, and do so in comparison to some relevant reference person known as a comparison other.[20]

An important addition to our understanding of organizational justice came when the concept of procedural justice was added to the literature. In simplest terms, procedural justice deals with one's perception of the fairness of the decision-making process.[21] As such, one may be dismayed by the distribution of outcomes, yet understand and accept the fundamental fairness of the way the distribution decision was made. Accordingly, perceptions of justice and fairness are maintained.

Let's consider an example. Carl Smith leads a 12-person department. The department exceeded its annual goals, allowing members to share in an attractive performance bonus. However, Smith felt, in the name of fairness, that one departmental member deserved an additional bump for the outstanding work and informal leadership he had provided during the past year. Smith made his case to the division manager, asking to dip into his discretionary merit money and support the hard-working employee with an additional 2 percent merit bump. The manager considered the request and asked to meet with Smith.

The manager agreed that the employee had an outstanding year and deserved every bit of the requested merit increase. But, without hesitation, the manager noted that he could not approve such an amount. He explained that two members of a different department had completed a high-profile project that had been more than two years in development. As such, the bulk of the discretionary merit money needed to go to them. Importantly, the logic seemed sound to Smith, and he even confided that if he were in the manager's chair, he would make the same decision. By explaining the process and reasoning behind his decision, the manager maintained the foundations of fairness.

It is rather alarming how infrequently managers take the time to convey the procedural logic. Justifications for this omission abound. "I'm paid to make the tough decisions," or, "I don't have time to justify every decision and appease every person." Or consider the understandable but all-too-frequent copout, "There are things I know that I cannot share." (Actually, that explanation, when it is the only valid explanation, carries positive weight in the context of fairness).

Let's dig a bit more deeply. Fair processes are characterized by decisions that are based on accurate information; are applied consistently; appear to be void of bias or vested interests; are consistent with prevailing standards of ethics and morality, and provide for the expression of concerns from those affected by the decisions.[22]

Consider one additional factor. When those affected by a decision are allowed to be actively involved in the decision-making process, in essence given a "voice," perceptions of procedural justice are enhanced.[23] While seemingly straightforward, this concept of voice is multilayered. While "authentic voice" has critical advantages, "inauthentic voice" can be a landmine that destroys perceptions of justice.

The difference between the two is strongly affected by perceptions of consideration. In short, when a leader requests employee input and employees oblige, these employees must believe that the leader is "actively considering" the input as decisions are made. Again, the most damning impact comes from perceptions of inauthentic voice: "He asked what I thought, but his mind was already made up."

Action Based in Respect

Warren Bennis was one of the most influential leadership thinkers of the past half century. Reflecting over his long career, Bennis concluded that the two most salient attributes of leaders are respect and trust.[24] We wholeheartedly agree. And most leaders probably concur. There is, however, a troubling complication. While the concepts of respect and trust are easy to espouse, they are rather tricky to enact and maintain. We have seen this in action, working with leaders who are sure they have created a tone of respect and trust, only to learn (often through the eye-popping clarity of 360-degree feedback) that others do not feel the same way. In the following sections, we will strive to make respect and trust become more than lofty concepts — mere words to be espoused. We will explore the behavioral dynamics necessary to make them live and impact your organizational context.

We recently worked with MaryAnn Brown, a clinician leader whose roles included leading some key quality initiatives. By our second meeting, we could already see that Brown was a passionate and concerned perfectionist who thrust herself into her work and expected the same of others. Her personal values echoed respect and trust, and she believed her interactions modeled these concepts. Both her work and her personal style could be characterized by one phrase — fast-paced.

Not surprisingly, Brown tended to be direct and unfiltered in her assessments of others and her directives about what should be done. She even argued that "facts are facts. I don't have time to sugarcoat everything." Fair enough, yet Brown seemed genuinely taken aback to learn that many people found her to be "cold, self-centered and disrespectful." What she espoused was not what was experienced.

There are two key building blocks of respect — significance and affirmation. Significance is both a perception and a feeling. Personal significance rises when people believe that they are important, they count, they make a difference and they are a "valued member of this organization."[25] People yearn for feelings of significance, and when experienced, it is a powerful motivator. We can help those around us feel the impact of their significance, or we can miss this key opportunity.

Significance begins to emerge when people feel that they are part of something important — that they are part of a "noble cause." In some industries, the quest for the noble cause may be elusive or hard to pinpoint. That is not the case with health care. The key is helping people realize that they are a valued component in the activity chain. For example, a blood draw is a basic technical task. Yet the impact on patient comfort, care and necessary analytics is indispensable. The technician needs to know and experience this noble cause.

To a large extent, significance is built through the second foundation — affirmation. Affirmation requires both recognizing and communicating to others credit and appreciation for the work they do. Physicians, often driven by high levels of inner motivation, may dismiss or discount the importance of overt expressions of affirmation. In simplest terms, most of us affirm too little and too infrequently.

Appropriate affirmations should take into account four considerations. First, affirmations should be seen as being earned and sincere. Blanket affirmations and unbridled praise (the oft-maligned "attaboys") have minimal impact and produce rapid satiation and may even have a boomerang effect when sincerity is questioned.

Second, affirmations should be perceived as realistic — consistent with the actions taken and the outcomes that have been attained. A simple statement of "thanks" tied directly to the desired outcome is often all that is necessary. "That was a tricky situation with that patient, and you handled it carefully, clearly and professionally. Thanks." It need not and should not be over-the-top.

Third, the affirmation should be timely. The reinforcement value and perceived impact will be higher if it is closely linked with the behavior and performance that is being recognized.

Fourth, and extremely important, the affirmation has its greatest impact when it comes from a credible source — someone who understands the value and effect of what has been done; someone who is close to the action; and someone who carries the respect that comes from expertise and authority. In many cases, that may be you.

Respect may also be understood by looking at its polar opposite — the damning impact of perceived disrespect. Certain behaviors undermine and destroy perceptions of respect. Some of these behaviors, such as bullying, intimidating and belittling, are overt and quite demonstrative. Others are more subtle, and they are drawn from the tone of communications and the nature of interpersonal interactions. These more subtle destroyers of respect occur when others conclude that you are self-centered, dismissive, arrogant and aloof, abrasive or negatively sarcastic. All are forms of interpersonal insensitivity.

We worked with too many leaders (physician and non-physician alike) who successfully control the direction of slowly paced meetings by clearly signaling their dissatisfaction and boredom through nonverbal diversionary tactics. As one leader noted, "When I get frustrated and have had enough, I turn to my cellphone, and people get the message pretty fast." While such actions may yield immediate results, they also plant seeds of disrespect. Alternative and more appropriate responses — such as orally summarizing, checking for clarity and encouraging the group to consider the next issue — are preferable.

Among all disrespectful behaviors, sarcasm is particularly nuanced. The use of dry, creative and at times humorous sarcasm is often the product of a bright and quick mind. It may be seen, in some circumstances, as a form of witty teasing that helps lighten the tone of a stress-laden workplace. The problem is that sarcasm is played out on a shifting context of fragile moods and feelings. What seemed like good-natured fun one day can be perceived as cruelty the next. In part, this is because of the insidious nature of sarcasm, a term that literally means to "rip and tear the flesh." A target may experience an episode of sarcasm as a form of personal diminution. Our advice, within the workplace context, is always the same: Given the risks involved, leaders are best served by avoiding expressions of workplace sarcasm.

There is one final behavioral twist worth noting. When people experience either disrespect or diminished significance, natural "fight or flight" tendencies are activated. Over time, self-confidence is affected. If prolonged, resentment and eventual disengagement are likely.

Foundations of Trust

Trust is a word that is bandied about, often without regard for context. It is the subject of broad oversimplification, and it is the vague menace behind a range of interactional ills. However, the concept has received considerable scholarly attention. Extensive research has portrayed the multifaceted nature of the term, as well as its tenuous and fragile nature. Importantly, we recognize that trust is built incrementally from shared experiences, and deep, meaningful trust requires regular interactions that can foster layers of understanding.

The centrality of trust is well established in the leadership literature, and an array of studies have helped us understand how trust affects outcomes ranging from employee loyalty and commitment to creativity and cooperation.[26] We have also gained a much clearer view of how trust is established and maintained.[27] In the process, we recognize that distrust in leadership (particularly immediate leadership) can lead to a series of dysfunctional results that include individual dissatisfaction, depleted motivation and eventual turnover. Finally, and especially important in today's fast-paced world, the existence of trust between parties may actually accelerate the interactive, decision-making process. This occurs, presumably, because less time is needed to independently verify the veracity of others' assertions.[28]

Like so many themes in the behavioral realm, trust is relationally driven. It involves a relationship between parties and is one of the attitudinal outcomes of that relationship. In short, trust is a belief that others can be relied on to do what they say they will do.[29] Trust always involves some level of risk — the risk of being vulnerable and the risk of losing control to another. Further, trust is built incrementally through direct experiences and face-to-face interactions. As such, trust is an attitude drawn from direct evidence formed from perceptions, beliefs and attributions about another party.[30]

Each of us has an idiosyncratic tendency to trust others largely drawn from our experiences. Those who have been burned by vesting trust in others are, reasonably, more likely to hold others at arm's length, demanding concrete interactive evidence before risking further trust. Others, with a series of positive trusting experiences, are likely to be more open, vulnerable and willing to extend trust. A caveat: The leader's trust is always being tested, constantly held to microscopic scrutiny. Behaviors, communications and words (or the lack thereof) carry real and symbolic messages that help shape others' perceptions of trust.

With this backdrop, let's look more deeply at how physician leaders can create a climate of trust. When one determines whether you are trustworthy, four key perceptual factors are considered: ability, benevolence, authenticity and consistency.[31]

Perceptions of ability arise when others believe that you have the skills, the competence and the capacity to carry through and do what you say you will do. Of course, these perceptions are context based. One may place complete trust in the physician's ability within a clinical context but question his ability in articulating broad personnel policies or directing strategic change. At times, leaders — full of bravado — promise outcomes (for example, a salary increase or a new assignment) where they do not have the authoritative capacity to deliver. Accordingly, ability to follow through becomes problematic in others' eyes.

Benevolence arises when those around you feel that your basic intent is to do what is good or right for them, the team and the broader organizational mission. In short, benevolence arises when you are perceived as being other-centered rather than self-centered. These perceptions are fundamentally judgments of character. Of course, perceptions of one's good intentions are drawn from the consideration, concern and sensitivity toward others that is displayed. The trick here is that others are inferring your underlying intention, at times with quite limited direct evidence.

Authenticity arises when leaders are seen as having deep convictions, core values and fundamental beliefs, and a willingness to behave so that there is consistency among these guiding principles and actions.[32] Perceptions of authenticity often hinge on what is called "relational transparency."[33] This involves being able to connect with others, letting them see and experience your true or core self. Of course, authentic leaders are willing to be vulnerable, and they are willing to display appropriate self-disclosure. Relational transparency rests on two assumptions: that there is a genuine connection between what we espouse and how we intend to act; and that we will be able to move beyond our emotional masks and express our views and feelings openly and honestly.

Consistency may be one of the most difficult factors for busy physicians. Perceptions of consistency are strongly affected by how we follow through on our commitments. With all good intention, we may promise an employee or colleague to "get back to you on that," only to falter from forgetfulness. Another common occurrence is the leader's promise to "check into it" — often a process that takes time as the issue at hand weaves its way through the structure of hierarchy and administrative handoffs. As time proceeds, it's easy for others to assume that you "dropped the ball" unless thoughtful and time-sensitive feedback check-ins are used. In any case, each incident of inconsistency can erode, at least to some extent, the base of perceived trust.

Leaders are always under the microscopic eye, with trust being earned and tested at each turn. What you say (and do not say), what you support (and refrain from supporting), and how you act (or do not act) all make powerful statements about trust. Like it or not, you deal with a sense of "leadership amplification." In other words, the things you do and say are amplified and seen by others as more important and meaningful than you ever imagined or intended. Here, little things mean a lot. An off-the-cuff comment, a lack of eye contact, a dismissive or perfunctory greeting as you enter a room, or a frown of disappointment may be magnified by others and perceived as a more significant message than you ever intended or realized.

Breaches of Trust

All leaders breach trust. There is no exception. In some cases, these breaches stem from intentional, malicious and egocentric moves that destroy relationships through calculated lies and manipulations. Sometimes, breaches arise as one gets caught in political complexities — providing a different version of events to different audiences in an attempt to either look better or at least look no worse. Dramatic and stinging as these occurrences can be, they are, in most organizational contexts, exceptions.

In their thoughtful book *Trust and Betrayal in the Workplace,* Dennis and Michelle Reina note that most of our breaches of trust are minor and unintentional.[34] Generally, they are acts of omission rather than commission. Yet these unintentional breaches can send powerful signals, dramatically impacting the impressions of those affected. Further, if such breaches are not addressed, they tend to fester and color future interactions. Make no mistake, failure to redress broken trust erodes the leader's credibility.

While we generally eschew formulaic approaches, a systematic framework for rebuilding these instances of damaged trust may be useful. The first step, "recognition and sensitivity," may be the most important. This step involves recognizing the potentially damaging nature of even minor breaches and grasping the significance of reaching out to offer remediation. Emotional perspective is important here. What may seem to be a small and rather benign oversight to you can (and probably will) be seen differently by the offended party.

Second, rebuilding and repairing broken trust demands a "personal meeting." While it is both tempting and convenient to turn to texts, emails or voicemail, these forms of technological connectivity are poor substitutes for the impact of face-to-face interactions. In general, when emotionally charged sensitivities are at play (as they are here), opt for direct and personal contact if at all possible.

Third, we suggest a quick "review of the issues" to make sure both parties understand the context and agree on the facts. Now comes the hard part.

The fourth step is to offer a "sincere apology for the part you played" in creating the breach of trust. Excuses and lengthy explanations get in the way at this stage, and they tend to diminish the impact of the apology. This need not be lengthy. "I should have checked with you before changing the protocol. That was unfair to you. I apologize."

It is reasonable at this point to expect the other party to express, perhaps with raised emotions, their concerns. The best course, generally, is to listen and validate the emotions that may be pouring out. At this point, it may be appropriate to explain your motives and the logic of your actions. Take ownership of the behavior that led to the breach. "You know, we had limited time, and I felt an immediate decision was needed. However, I should have made an effort to reach out to you, and I did not."

The final stage is what we call "the future." Here, you assert intentions and behavioral commitments for the future. "My intention is to keep you involved. Unless it is completely impractical, I will do so in the future." Part of this step may be include working with the other party to determine how future complicating issues can be best handled. Of course, time and consistency of action will determine the extent of the rebuilding efforts. Recall that trust is built incrementally, over time. Similarly, how it is rebuilt incrementally, over time, is hopefully through a series of successive actions that demonstrate consistency of intent.

Emotional Intelligence

Conceptions and definitions of emotional intelligence (EI) come from a range of sources and provide considerable variation. Broadly, EI may be conceived as "the set of abilities (verbal and nonverbal) that enable a person to generate, recognize, express, understand and evaluate their own and others' emotions in order to guide thinking and action that successfully cope with environmental demands and actions."[35]

Although themes of EI have appeared in the behavioral literature for years, the construct gained broad interest and more focused attention with the publication of Daniel Goleman's 1995 bestseller, *Emotional Intelligence: Why It Can Matter More Than IQ.*[36] Subsequent empirical investigations have offered mixed outcomes, and the EI construct has fostered an array of support and criticism. The efficacy of key components is not generally at issue, but rather the overall predictive capacity of the emotional intelligence construct.

More specifically, concern seems to focus on hyperbolic claims, such as the oft-quoted phrase, "For those in leadership positions, emotional intelligence skills account for close to 90 percent of what distinguishes outstanding leaders from those judged as average.[37] In short, we recognize the importance of EI but need the clarity of perspective.

Recent empirical efforts are promising. For example, meta-analyses have shown a positive and significant relationship between EI and overall job performance.[38] Further, a meta-analysis of 20 studies involving more than 5,000 participants found a significant positive relationship between EI and constructive conflict management, arguably one of the more critical components of leadership.[39] As such, since emotional and relational qualities are important to leader success, the absence of EI competencies can inhibit a leader's growth and progress.[40]

Perhaps most critical within this discussion is the realization that EI is neither innate nor fixed. The skills and competencies of EI can be developed and enhanced. Of course, as with any skill development, focused attention, guidance (often aided by coaching) and ongoing practice is required.

With this background, let's explore three of the more critical competencies or behaviors within EI, along with related applications — all with a careful eye on the unique challenges facing physician leaders.

Emotional Self-Awareness

Most models agree that emotional self-awareness is the foundation of EI. This competency deals with our ability to be in touch with our feelings, moods and overall emotional state and understand how the display of these emotions affects others. At least three interconnected factors are at play here. First, we must be aware of our personal emotional state. Second, we must understand why these emotions occur. Third, we must be able to read and recognize how the presence of our emotions impacts those around us.

Not surprisingly, leaders with high levels of emotional self-awareness are "attuned to their inner signals."[41] They have developed the capacity to recognize emerging emotions (perhaps frustration, disappointment or anger) as they arise.

One physician shared with us, "When my expectations are not met, I am almost always immediately disappointed. I can sense myself getting agitated and nervous. I try as hard as I can to mask this, but others seem to read me like a book, and they quickly assume that I am mad." Here, self-awareness (and more specifically, awareness of the interactive pattern that unfolds) provided the leader with a powerful set of possibilities. When asked if the inferred designation of "mad" was indeed accurate, he hedged. "Sure, sometimes, but usually not — I am really just frustrated and disappointed."

Armed with this awareness, the leader can label his emotions rather than allow others to draw more extreme interpretations. For example, an open and honest statement such as "I am disappointed with these results" could help establish a more appropriate perspective.

Emotion Regulation

Emotion regulation refers to "the process by which individuals influence which emotions they have, when they have them, and how they experience and express these emotions."[42] Since emotion regulation is the means for creating and sustaining positive affective states, we accept that it is logically related to job performance.[43] For example, followers both desire and expect their leaders to project optimism and resiliency, and the expression of these emotions and moods is particularly acute during times of change and stress.[44]

Emotion regulation has another side. Here, we focus on the skill of emotional self-control or what has popularly been known as impulse control. Pioneering EI researcher Reuven Bar-On describes impulse control as "the ability to resist or delay an impulse, drive or temptation to act ... or to react appropriately without uncontrolled anger."[45] Not surprisingly, the lack of appropriate impulse control is one of the major reasons that leaders derail from a trajectory of leader advancement.[46]

Recently, researchers have suggested a cascading model of EI, where emotion perception, emotion understanding and emotion regulation emerge in a progressive manner.[47] There is merit and innate logic to this approach. In other words, emotion perception precedes emotion understanding, which in turn leads to conscious acts of emotion regulation.[48]

Let's probe these themes a bit. Recently, we worked with a surgical specialty center that brought us in contact with Dr. Groves and his staff. Groves, as both a talented surgeon and a physician leader, fostered an interactive tone that ranged from conciliation and concern to anger and rage — all depending on his mood. His flares of anger were so extreme that his nurses would at times prompt patients not to be offended by the doctor's occasional terse and derisive tone. The nurses would attempt to lessen the sting by suggesting, "This is just how he is today."

Working with Groves, we faced some polarized possibilities. First, it was possible that he simply did not realize how he was coming across and affecting others — an issue of emotional self-awareness. Second, perhaps he did possess such awareness and just did not care. Or third, it was possible that he recognized the impact but found he was unable to curb his intensity given the pressure and time-sensitive nature of his work. Of course, both the second and third explanations raise concerns of emotion regulation.

Working with Groves, it seemed that all three possible explanations were at play. Although Groves was acutely aware of his tendency to "get annoyed" with others, he did not seem to recognize the dramatic impact this had on those around him. In turn, he saw little need to more carefully regulate his expressions. Interestingly, but not surprisingly, Groves engaged his peers and administrators the way he did his staff. At times, he was warm and understanding. At other times, he was overly demanding, unwilling to yield on any position to which he had committed, and abusive.

Dealing with issues of destructive and diminished emotional self-control is a tricky task. Recognizing the interpersonal impact is important. Sensing early signals of rising emotional intensity is also key. Developing a series of appropriate diversionary tactics to help thwart an emotional outburst can be helpful.

For example, we often encourage those who get frustrated during lengthy meetings and burst forward with statements they wish they could retract to try a three-step process: Become sensitive to early signals of rising emotional intensity (that nervous sensation or the shaking leg); divert your energies to appropriate outlets (perhaps write down what you are thinking of saying), and, through the first two steps, carefully assess whether to act. In the name of transparency, while Groves is developing, he remains a work in progress.

In Warren Bennis' memoir of his life in leadership, he speaks of his admiration and respect for an early mentor, Douglas McGregor. McGregor, known for his "Theory X and Theory Y assumptions" about individual attitudes toward work, was an educational pioneer and an original thought leader who helped crystalize the significance of the human factor at work.

Bennis spoke of McGregor's tone — his character and his interpersonal manner.

"One of his MIT colleagues pointed out that he (McGregor) had a rare ability 'to absorb punishment.' That sounded like a questionable virtue, but it was a genuine strength — one that serves leaders well and one that few leaders have. He never flinched, at least in public, no matter how unflatteringly people spoke to or about him. Instead, he seemed energized by criticism, as if the clash of opinions was more valuable than consensus, however comfortable consensus might be." [49]

So what does all of this mean? Recall that emotional intelligence can be learned. Sensitivities can be enhanced, and a lack of emotional regulation and impulse control can be curbed.

Empathy

Displaying empathy and understanding has long been considered one of the behavioral factors that differentiate thriving from struggling leaders.[50] Cambridge University professor Simon Baron-Cohen defines empathy as "the ability to identify what someone else is thinking or feeling and to respond to that person's thoughts and feelings with an appropriate emotion."[51]

Within this context, Daniel Goleman has added further refinement and clarity. In a recent work, Goleman argues that empathy should not be viewed as a single attribute. Rather, he presents three distinct kinds of empathy: cognitive empathy — "the ability to understand another person's perspective"; emotional empathy — "the ability to feel what someone else feels"; and empathic concern — "the ability to sense what another person needs from you."[52] Each of these kinds of empathy offers special challenges worthy of deeper exploration.

Cognitive empathy — the ability to grasp and understand another's point of view — is often clouded by our deep commitment to our own point of view, a behavioral tendency known as the commitment bias.[53] Interestingly, as we study and gain expertise in a subject, our commitment to our perspective, our commitment bias, becomes deeper and stronger. Not surprisingly, this commitment bias may lead us to diminish or dismiss arguments and views that differ from our preconceived understanding of the issue. Accordingly, difficulty in understanding another's perspective may be intensified.

Emotional empathy has its own unique complications. For example, some researchers have suggested that physicians learn (beginning with medical school training) to block their impulse to empathize with others' feelings in order to make less emotional, more objective and ultimately better decisions.[54] Such emotional control seems quite appropriate in some contexts and less so in others. Further, when applied and practiced repeatedly, one may experience a depleted appreciation for emotional empathy.

Empathic concern requires emotional sensitivity that has a unique action-focused perspective. Sensing what another needs within a given context is always nuanced and subject to misinterpretation. As successful achievers, physicians tend to be "fixers" — quickly capable of assessing the situation and moving toward premeditative action. In many contexts, others might prefer that we listen rather than fix. We will expand on this theme in the next chapter.

What We Say and What We Do

In his seminal work on organizational culture, Edgar Schein distinguished between the espoused culture and the real or enacted culture.[55] The espoused culture represents who we "say" we are — the values, orientations and be-havioral outcomes that are desired. The real culture represents what actually "is" — the themes and values that we live, that are practiced day to day, and that are reinforced and rewarded. While we can espouse wonderful cultural values, the more critical concern is whether they are real, and whether they are enacted through the behaviors of our people.

The leadership extension is clear. Leaders may espouse lofty rhetoric that is consistent with generally accepted best practices. Yet we wonder — are those themes modeled? Are they practiced? Are they expected and rewarded? Are they real? In the past, we have read to our students the final portion of a university commencement address that was delivered by a prominent corpo-rate CEO. He lauded the principle of fairness, the foundational grounding of solid business ethics, and the constant drive to assure that our competitive zeal never destroyed our integrity and humanity. Less than two weeks later, he was indicted for insider trading. The students were left to ponder the cul-tural implications of what was real and what was merely espoused.

We work with leaders throughout the world. They represent a range of organizations and industries. With few exceptions, these leaders espouse a surprisingly consistent set of core values — quality, respect, integrity, trust, customer focus and an inherent commitment to their most important asset, their people. They herald the significance of giving people a voice and lis-tening to their concerns; open and transparent communication; fairness and justice; and soliciting and considering input before decisions are made. Their pronouncements are often delivered with a moving and masterful passion.

However, when the leader's words are viewed through a different lens — the lens of those who are touched and impacted by the leader's actions — a divergent version of reality may emerge. And, of course, most people conclude that what we do as leaders (as opposed to what we say) is a far more valid insight into who we are as leaders. Leadership authorities Jim Kouzes and Barry Posner have pushed leaders to "model the way" — in essence, being a visible example to others by acting in concert with what they espouse.[56] Leadership pioneer Warren Bennis expressed the same thought: "Everything the leader does reflects what he or she is."[57]

These points seem so obvious, yet they are so often missed. At times, as we work with physician leaders, we have the opportunity to observe them in their clinical settings. On a recent visit with one leader, we walked with him through the clinic halls toward his office. During the brief walk, we encountered one of the physician's nurses. We stopped, and I stood shyly aside as he berated her for not having the proper supplies available in one of the patient rooms. The one-sided exchange was pointed and public. Later, as I left, I encountered the nurse, obviously still stinging from embarrassment. She commented to me, "You know he's just a perfectionist. We don't take it personally."

Really? I wondered what was being modeled. I questioned why high standards could not be achieved by less offensive means. I wondered what sort of temperament the patient experienced as the doctor reached into the drawer and failed to find what he expected and needed.

I reminded myself that the physician's work was time sensitive and stressful; that errors carry unthinkable costs; and that as an outsider I was viewing only a small segment of a larger interpersonal pattern. Yet I also knew that what I had just experienced was part of a pattern that played out in unfortunate and inappropriate exchanges with fellow physicians and administrators — which was precisely why we had begun to meet!

There is a deeper and more insidious consideration here. Whenever there is a disconnect between what we espouse and how we behave, a set of interrelated behavioral processes come into play.

First, others begin to question our authenticity. Author and former CEO Bill George candidly noted, "I believe that leadership begins and ends with authenticity."[58] While considerable research and study has explored the nature of authenticity, some ideas are central. Authenticity hinges on three factors: "core self-awareness" — the ability to understand and center on your core personal values; "value consistency" — the ability to exercise emotional regulation and self-control so that our actual behavior is in line with our core values, and "relational transparency" — the ability to allow others to see and experience your core self.

Concluding Thoughts: The Art of Finesse

As a young professor, I had the opportunity to work on some challenging organizational projects that were led by a senior professor of economics, Doug Thorson. Thorson was a curious and well-published intellectual with a pragmatic approach to people and groups. He always strove for inclusion, even when my immature eyes thought we were extending consideration much too far. Although Thorson could be direct and adamantly decisive, I never saw him behave toward others dismissively, derisively or disrespectfully. He recognized and extended appreciation for divergent views. Although I am sure he experienced his share of interpersonal frustrations, I never saw him raise his voice or display anger toward another.

But the quality I respected most and sought most deeply to understand and emulate was his unflappable tendency to be able to work every situation to advance our team goals. Thorson was a keen observer of people, a careful purveyor of political undertones and a guru of reading and assessing the situational dynamics at hand — and he did it all seamlessly and naturally. To sum up his style in one word, Thorson had *finesse*.

I find myself returning to the word finesse as I work with physician leaders. "You can come at it that way, but the risks seem high. Perhaps you need to finesse that a bit." At times, this advice is viewed as an act of capitulation, and the receiving party plows ahead, guns blazing. Often, this style yields an immediate victory and a legacy of tone that haunts and alters future interactions — rarely for the better.

Finesse is not capitulation. It is leadership. Finesse may be viewed as a skill or set of skills that help one to handle sensitive and challenging encounters resourcefully and adroitly. It involves reading the situation, the people, the pressures, the politics and the needs that are all spinning with mysterious confluence. Finesse demands an understanding and use of the formidable interpersonal dynamics we have developed in this chapter. At times, finesse becomes a form of personal self-talk and quick but well-reasoned internal deliberation. As such, "I say what's on my mind" is replaced with "I don't have to say everything I think." "I tell it like it is" becomes "How will this be received?" And, "I know what's best" becomes "How can we get others on board?"

The art of finesse rests on grasping the fundamental needs that are at the heart of interpersonal exchanges. In their classic work on negotiation, *Getting to Yes,* Roger Fisher, William Ury and Bruce Patton assert that "demands come from unmet needs." It is one of those statements that is profound in its simplicity. We will dig more deeply into this area in the next chapter as we probe the dynamics of successful dialogue.

1. Goleman, D; Boyatzis, R. & McKee, A. (2002). *Primal Leadership: Realizing the power of emotional intelligence.* Boston: Harvard Business School Press, p. 3.

2. Mast, M.S.; Jonas, K.; Cronauer, C.K.; & Darioly, A. (2012). On the importance of the superior's interpersonal sensitivity for good leadership. *Journal of Applied Social Psychology, 42*(5), 1043-1068.

3. Ibid.

4. Hall, J.A. (1984). *Nonverbal Sex Differences: Communication accuracy and expressive style.* Baltimore: Johns Hopkins University Press. McClure, E.B. (2000). A meta-analytic review of sex differences in facial expression processing and their development in infants, children, and adolescents, *Psychological Bulletin, 126,* 424-453.

5. Beer, M. & Nohria, N. (2000). Cracking the code of change. *Harvard Business Review,* 78(3), 133-141. Karp, T. & Helgo, T.I.T. (2009). Reality revisited: Leading people in chaotic change. *Journal of Management Development,* 28(2), 81-93.

6. Heath, C. & Heath, D. (2010). *Switch: How to change when change is hard.* New York: Broadway Books.

7. Van Buren, M. & Safferstone, T. (2009). The quick wins paradox. *Harvard Business Review,* 87(1), 54-61. McCall Jr.; Lombardo, M.W.; & Morrison, A.M. (1998). *Lessons of Experience: How successful executives develop on the job.* Lexington, MA: Lexington Books.

8. Gladwell, M. (2005). *Blink: The power of thinking without thinking.* New York: Little Brown.

9. Levinson, W.; Roter, D.L.; Mullooly, J.P.; Dull, V.T.; & Frankel, R.M. (1997). Physician-patient communication: The relationship with malpractice claims among primary care physicians and surgeons. *Journal of the American Medical Association, 277,* 553-559.

10. Goleman, D; Boyatzis, R. & McKee, A. (2002). *Primal Leadership: Realizing the power of emotional intelligence.* Boston: Harvard Business School Press.

11. Ibid., p. 8.

12. Ibid., p. 8.

13. Horine, K.R. (2015). Taking the lead. *Kentucky Monthly, 18*(1), 36-39.

14. Adams, J.S. (1965). Inequity in social exchange. In L. Berkowitz (Ed.), *Advances in Experimental and Social Psychology* (Vol. 2, pp. 267-299). New York: Academic Press. Weick, K.E. (1967). The concept of equity in the perception of pay. *Administrative Science Quarterly, 2,* 414-439.

15. Cohen-Charash, Y. & Spector, P.E. (2001). The role of justice in organizations: A meta-analysis. *Organizational Behavior and Human Decision Processes, 86*(2), 278-321. Colquitt, J.A.; Conlon, D.E.; Wesson, M.J.; Porter, C.O.L.H.; & Ng, K.Y. (2001). Justice at the millennium: A meta-analaytic review of 25 years of organizational justice research. *Journal of Applied Psychology, 86*(3), 425-445.

16. Li, A. & Cropanzano, R. (2009). Do East Asians respond more/less strongly to organizational justice than North Americans? *Journal of Management Studies, 46*(5), 787-805.

17. Ibid, p. 789-790.

18. Colquitt, *et al.,* 2001.

19. Nowakowski, J.M. & Conlon, D.E. (2005). Organizational justice: Looking back, looking forward. *The International Journal of Conflict Management, 16*(1), 4-29, p. 5.

20. Adams, 1965.

21. Nowakowski & Conlon, 2005.

22. Leventhal, G.S.; Karuza, J. & Fry, W.R. (1980). Beyond fairness: A theory of allocation preferences. In G. Mikula (Ed.), *Justice and Social Interaction* (pp. 167-218). New York: Springer-Verlag.

23. Thibaut, J.W. & Walker, L. (1975). *Procedural Justice: A psychological perspective.* Hillsdale, N.J.: Erlbaum.

24. Bennis, W. (2014). Respect and trust: The two most salient attributes of leaders. *Leadership Excellence,* 11-12.

25. Burchell, M. & Robin, J. (2011). *The Great Workplace: How to build it, how to keep it, and why it matters.* San Francisco: Jossey-Bass, p. 17.

26. Aryee, L.S. & West, S.G. (2002). Trust as a mediator of the relationship between organizational justice and organizational outcomes: Test of a social exchange model. *Journal of Organizational Behavior,* 23, 267-285. Zalabak, P.S.; Ellis, K.; & Winograd, G. (2000). Organizational Trust: What it means and why it matters. *Organizational Development Journal,* 18, 35-49. Zhang, A.Y.; Tsui, A.S.; Song, L.J.; & Jia, L. (2008). How do I trust thee? The employee-organization relationship, supervisory support and middle manager trust in the organization. *Human Resource Management,* 47(1), 111-132.

27. Galford, R. & Drapeau, A.S. (2003). The enemies of trust. *Harvard Business Review,* 81(2), 88-95. Perry, R.W., & Mankin, L.D. (2004). Understanding employee trust in management: Conceptual clarification and correlates. *Public Personnel Management,* 33(3), 277-290. Tan, H.H., & Lim, A.K. (2009). Trust in coworkers and trust in organizations. *The Journal of Psychology,* 143(1), 45-66.

28. Covey, S.M.R. (2006). The Speed of Trust: The One Thing That Changes Everything. New York: Free Press.

29. McCauley, C.D.; Moxley, R.S.; & Van Velsor, E. (Eds.). (1998). *Handbook of Leadership Development.* San Francisco: Jossey-Bass.

30. Tan & Lim, 2009.

31. Mayer, R.C.; Davis, J.H.; & Schoorman, F.D. (1995). An integrative model of organizational trust. *Academy of Management Review,* 20, 709-734.

32. Walumba, F.O.; Avolio, B.; Gardner, W.; Wernsing, T.; & Peterson, S. (2008). Authentic leadership: Development of a theory-based measure. *Journal of Management,* 34(1), 89-126.33.

34. Avolio, B.J. & Gardner, W.L. (2005). Authentic leadership development: Getting to the root of positive forms of leadership. *The Leadership Quarterly,* 16, 315-338.

35. Reina, D.S. & Reina, M.L. (2006). *Trust and Betrayal in the Workplace.* San Francisco: Berrett-Koehler.

36. Van Rooy, D. & Viswesvaran, C. (2004). Emotional intelligence: A meta-analytic investigation of predictive validity and nomological net. *Journal of Vocational Behavior,* 65, 71-95, p.72.

37. Goleman, D. (1995). *Emotional Intelligence: Why it can matter more than IQ.* New York: Bantam Books.

38. Kemper, C. L. (1999). EQ vs. IQ. *Communication World,* 16, 15-22, p. 16. Lindebaum, D. (2009). Rhetoric or remedy: A critique on developing emotional intelligence. *Academy of Management Learning & Education,* 8, 225-237.

39. O'Boyle, Jr., E.H.; Humphrey, R.H.; Pollack, J.M.; Hawver, T.H.; & Story, P.A. (2011). The relation between emotional intelligence and job performance: A meta-analysis. *Journal of Organizational Behavior,* 32, 788-818. Van Rooy, D. & Viswesvaran, C. (2004). Emotional intelligence: A meta-analytic investigation of predictive validity and nomological net. *Journal of Vocational Behavior,* 65, 71-95.

40. Schlaerth, A.; Ensari, N.; & Christian, J. (2013). A meta-analytic review of the relationship between emotional intelligence and leaders' constructive conflict management. *Group Processes & Intergroup Relations,* 16(1), 126-136.

41. Goleman, D. (1998). *Working with Emotional Intelligence.* New York: Bantam Books.

42. Goleman, D.; Boyatzis, R.; & McKee, A. (2002). *Primal Leadership: Realizing the power of emotional intelligence.* Boston: Harvard Business School Press.

43. Gross, J.J. (1998). The emerging field of emotion regulation: An integrative review. *Review of General Psychology,* 2, 271-299.

44. Joseph, D.L. & Newman, D.A. (2010). Emotional intelligence: An Integrative meta-analysis and cascading model. *Journal of Applied Psychology,* 95(1), 54-78.45.

46. Goleman, 2002.

47. Bar-On, R. (2002). *The Emotional Quotient Inventory.* North Towanda, NY: Multi-Help Systems, p. 18.

48. Leslie, J.B. (2003). *Leadership Skills and Emotional Intelligence.* Greensboro, NC: The Center for Creative Leadership.

49. Joseph, D.L. & Newman, D.A. (2010). Emotional intelligence: An Integrative meta-analysis and cascading model. *Journal of Applied Psychology,* 95(1), 54-78. Mayer, J.D. & Salovey, P. (1997). What is emotional intelligence. In P. Salovey & D. Sluyter (Eds.), *Emotional Development and Emotional Intelligence: Implications for educators* (pp. 3-34). New York: Basic Books.

50. Joseph & Newman, 2010.

51. Bennis, W. (2010). *Still Surprised: A memoir of a life in leadership.* San Francisco: Jossey-Bass, p. 43.

52. Van Buren, M. & Safferstone, T. (2009). The quick wins paradox. *Harvard Business Review,* 87(1), 54-61.

53. Baron-Cohen, S. (2011). The empathy bell curve. *Phi Kappa Phi Forum,* 91(1), 10-12, p. 10.

54. Goleman, D. (2013). The focused leader. *Harvard Business Review,* 91(12), 50-60, p. 55.

55. Staw, B.M. (1976). Knee-deep in the big muddy: A study of escalating commitment to a chosen course of action. *Organizational Behavior and Human Performance,* 16(1), 27-44.

56. Goleman, 2013.

57. Schein, E.H. (2010). *Organizational Culture and Leadership* (4th ed.). San Francisco: Jossey-Bass.

58. Kouzes, J.M. & Posner, B.Z. (2002). *The Leadership Challenge.* San Francisco: Jossey-Bass.

59. Bennis, W. (2003). *On Becoming a Leader.* Cambridge, MA: Perseus Publishing.

60. George, W.W. (2003). *Authentic Leadership: Rediscovering the secrets to creating lasting value.* San Francisco: Jossey-Bass, p. 11.

4

Dialogue: Communicating for Understanding and Influence

··

OVER THE PAST 25 YEARS, WE HAVE WORKED WITH THOUSANDS OF leaders and have coached hundreds. These talented leaders have come from varied contexts, and each has exhibited a unique personality, perspective and approach. Some were ready for the leadership challenge and some were not. Some soared and others struggled. We have celebrated successes and carefully dissected outcomes that fell short of expectations.

Through it all, one theme affirmed by an array of researchers has emerged: Interpersonal communication is a fundamental differentiator between leader success and failure.[1] Some experts have taken an additional step, asserting that communication is the most important skill for overall career success.[2] And, there is every reason to believe that these conclusions are applicable to the roles you pursue. For example, in a survey of physician leaders, physician educators and medical students, researchers found that "interpersonal and communication skills" were central to effective physician leadership.[3]

When carried out effectively, the leaders' communications convey direction and purpose, thus aligning people and providing points of focus during periods of change and uncertainty. Effective leader communications enable others to have "voice," thereby engaging people across boundaries in important decisions that enhance the chances of securing needed outcomes.[4] Leader communication, when engaged openly and positively, builds rapport, emboldens trust, improves decision quality, increases acceptance and helps to ensure successful implementation of prescribed actions.

Of course, there is another side. At times, a leader's creative and promising initiatives crumble. Discussions get heated and egos get bruised. Teams that are populated with talented and dedicated people may splinter into camps with each pursuing divergent and self-serving agendas. Superficial collaboration replaces in-depth dialogue, eroding trust and creating cautious and fear-driven interactions.

We all realize that interpersonal and organizational problems such as these are rarely one-dimensional, and it's generally dangerous to think in terms of single causality. However, these unfortunate experiences and outcomes generally share a commonality — nonexistent, underused or poorly applied interpersonal communications.

Consider, for example, a recent study, drawn from a series of in-depth interviews with senior human resource managers. Here, researchers found that interpersonal communication skills (including areas such as active listening, message clarity and collaborative tone) were the skill areas where managers were most deficient.[5]

Leaders spend a surprising 80 percent of the typical work-day involved in various forms of communication.[6] Even more striking, evidence indicates that 81 percent of top-level communication takes place face to face and generally involves only a few people.[7] Among executives, about 60 percent of this communication is focused on listening.[8] About 14 percent of the leader's communication efforts fail — succumbing to a variety of preventable breakdowns.[9]

As a clinician, you entered the world of leadership with unique background and perspective. Through experience, you have ideas and evidence about what works and what does not. Accepting the challenge of leadership, you have committed to meld your formidable expertise and talent with the varied perspectives of others, focusing collectively and collaboratively on the organization's competitive progress. Along the way, you probably have encountered some recalcitrant colleagues, a few confusing political entanglements and some dramatic environmental challenges that demand action — all contained within an organizational context where the pace of progress may seem to be glacial at best. Each of these concerns begs for deeper and more effective interpersonal communication.

We have written elsewhere about the "under-communication bias," an alarming tendency among many leaders.[10] Here, while leaders understand the critical nature of communication, they communicate far too little, generally out of a fear of communicating too much. The paradox of the under-communication bias arises from a series of flawed, albeit well-intentioned assumptions. Sifting through these complexities, most under-communication occurs because we do not want to bog down busy people with too much information, we fear being labeled as a "micro-manager" and we assume that others are like us — motivated self-starters who neither need nor desire excessive guidance.[11]

While it is true that most leaders faced with fast-paced, high-stress, rapid-change contexts tend to communicate less rather than more, this is precisely the opposite of what is needed at the personal and interpersonal level.[12] There is considerable merit to the adage that during times of stress and change, it is virtually impossible to communicate too much. Further, when change occurs and tensions rise, people tend to fill in communication gaps with their own "inventions of understanding" — leading to dangerous rumors and unnecessary resistance.

With all these perspectives in mind, let's dig more deeply into some of the important interpersonal communication themes. This chapter provides a unique look at creating reciprocal understanding through deep listening, respectful inquiry, open-ended questioning and engaged dialogue. Our goal is building understanding and influence through meaningful collaborative exchanges.

Reciprocal Understanding

Communication may be viewed as the transfer of information and understanding from one party to another. The simplicity of this definition belies the complexity of actually making it happen. For example, the transfer of information — moving messages from one party to another — has never had more options or more opportunities for breakdown. Understanding is even more nuanced. Even when data are received, personal feelings, needs and vested interests enter the mix and complicate interpretations.

In his bestseller *The 7 Habits of Highly Successful People,* Stephen Covey offers straightforward insights. "Seek first to understand ... diagnose before (you) prescribe."[13] Indeed, reciprocal understanding — where each party sincerely seeks to understand the other — can change the tone of interpersonal exchanges.

However, there is an important complication to reciprocal understanding.

Reciprocal understanding involves grasping the "understory," which is rich in complexity, flavored by personal nuance. Words and messages are what we see and hear. The understory lies beneath the surface, ripe with emotional impact. While the understory may be difficult to share and often remains unexpressed, it drives behavior.

Consider the following example. As part of an earlier research project, one of the authors interviewed working parents of children with autism.[14] When asked what their colleagues at work knew of their family situation, the parents noted that most peers possessed a cursory awareness at best. "They know we have a child with special needs, and some know that he has autism."

Listening thoughtfully to the stories of these parents, a powerful understory emerged. They spoke of the struggle to attain a diagnosis. They described the wrenching realization that a traditional, idealized family dynamic would never be part of their lives. They addressed their battles to receive services. They described commonplace events like a trip to the dentist or the grocery store as emotional juggernauts. And they spoke of amazing sacrificial love for their children. They spoke of their willingness to fight for their children in a culture that misunderstood and often preferred to dismiss the needs and rights of their children.

To a person, these parents spoke of the significance of their work; their commitment to their organizations; and, above all, their unwavering commitment that their child's needs would take precedence over their job when necessary. In short, the understory affected everything. And the understory was generally untapped and unrealized by workplace peers.

For most organizational members, our understories are less dramatic. Or are they?

The Logic of Engaged Listening

We were not surprised to hear that Jared Brown had been asked to serve in a key leadership position within his health care system. As a primary care physician, Brown was well liked and highly respected. Patients appreciated his conversational style. While keeping a focused eye on the diagnostic results, he gleaned special insights by engaging his patients, carefully listening as their stories emerged, asking penetrating questions for clarity and depth of understanding. He seemed to create a masterful blend of both personal and data-driven evidence.

In his new administrative role, Brown applied the same open and calming approach to his new colleagues — other physician leaders, business-focused administrators and key team members from clinical and nonclinical backgrounds. One non-clinician summed up Brown's interpersonal approach succinctly. "He listens and he asks the right questions. As a result, when he weighs in, people pay attention."

From all appearances, Brown used the skills of engaged listening and expansive questioning — skills that are the foundational links for interpersonal communication. But these skills can be difficult to master within the complex maze of interpersonal dynamics. Further, these skills are even more difficult to maintain, especially when confronted with blocking, argumentative team members and time-sensitive needs.

We use the term *engaged listening* to emphasize the active nature and relational depth of this approach. The term also provides a clear distinction from the more common superficial listening, often referred to as mindless listening, that seems to inundate many organizational contexts.[15] You live and work in a high-pressure, fast-paced environment. You are bombarded by messages, most of which are irrelevant, deserving scant attention and ready dismissal. As such, tendencies toward superficial listening may have developed through the habit of necessity. In fact, the term *expansive questioning* is used to draw contrast to the more closed and limited nature of many "facts-only" approaches. Let's look at the difference-making approach of engaged listening in more depth.

The Dynamics of Engaged Listening

We have all seen the listener, fidgeting in his seat, just waiting for the speaker to take a breath so he can enter the fray. We are reminded of the piercing sarcasm of the commentary, "Are you really listening or just getting ready to talk?" Armed with this image, let's explore the five essential themes of engaged listening that are summarized here.

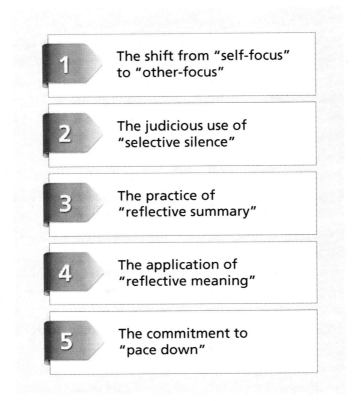

1	The shift from "self-focus" to "other-focus"
2	The judicious use of "selective silence"
3	The practice of "reflective summary"
4	The application of "reflective meaning"
5	The commitment to "pace down"

Table 4.1 — The Five Essential Themes of Engaged Listening

Engaged listening begins with a shift from self-focus to other-focus. Kenneth Cloke and Joan Goldsmith offer insight as they note, "Effective listening does not actually start with listening, rather it begins when the listener clears the decks and focuses his or her undivided attention on the person who is about to speak."[16]

Daniel Goleman refers to the same process as "attunement." "We offer a person our total attention and listen fully. We seek to understand the other person rather than just making our own point."[17]

This shift in focus or perspective may be the most complicated and least applied aspect of the process of engaged listening. Four other-focus demands: that we really do care about the other party's views; that we truly believe others have valuable views to offer; that we want to hear and understand what ideas they are conveying, and that we recognize that engaged listening is the precursor to learning from the contributions of others are key.

The intentionality of this mindset must be augmented by behavioral cues, most of which are expressed nonverbally. This is what others see. Eye contact, active facial expressions, periodic gestures of understanding and even a smile convey focused attention to the speaker. These expressions also connote respect, interest and a desire to work collaboratively.

A tinge of reality is needed. We recently worked with a physician leader, struggling mightily as he worked with a key, cross-functional team. Listening and dissecting a series of exchanges that the physician reported, we offered our thoughts on other-focused assumptions and actions. Receiving our input, he paused thoughtfully for a moment or two. "Yeah, but I really don't value what they have to say."

While his honesty was rather commendable, the limit of his leadership range was palpable. Despite a broad range of talent at the table, the team would advance no farther and no faster than the range of this physician's talents. Further, the dismissive nature of his assumptions were likely felt by all in attendance. In today's dynamic climate, such approaches to leadership are limiting. They simply are not good enough.

There is another deterrent to other-focused listening: the demon of multi-tasking. Recent research has confirmed what many of us suspected: Multi-tasking is relatively ineffective and highly inefficient. A colleague may have said it best: "It's a chance to screw up a lot of things at once." Of course, your clinical world demands accessibility, and others, for the most part, understand and accept this. Engaged listening, however, is and must be a decidedly mono-tasking activity.

Before leaving the theme of engaged listening, a few subtleties must be noted. For years, it has been the custom of my wife and me to sit on our porch in the evening, share a glass of wine and unwind our days for each other. As an introvert and one quite sensitive to maintaining the confidentiality of my coaching clients, I offer brief blurbs and snippets of my day. She, on the other hand, is a wonderfully open and expressive woman. Like many of you reading this book, I am also a problem solver. Consequently, as my wife explains a tricky or bothersome situation, I do what I do best. I launch into my "solve it" mode. One evening, as I began to unravel her situation, she intervened and drew my well-intended talk to a halt. "No, would you just shut up and listen?" Point made and taken.

Indeed, one of the most powerful forms of engaged listening can be "selective silence." Here, we listen intently. We offer nonverbal cues (eye contact, body posture and affirming movements) to denote our interest and focus. Yet we need not jump in with an immediate response. Selective silence can indicate to the other party that we have indeed focused on his or her agenda. Further, when used judiciously, it can encourage the speaker to probe more deeply, perhaps reaching richer awareness and self-discovered solutions. Above all, in cases where strong emotions are being expressed, it is the most respectful form of response. We are reminded of what most successful leadership coaches know and apply: "Often, less is more."

Selective silence is most effective when paired with "reflective summary." The reflective summary response occurs as we reflect back or express to the other party what we have just heard and learned. This is the tangible signal to the other party that he or she has been heard. Importantly, the reflective summary is factually oriented rather than interpretive. "Let me see if I have heard you. There seem to be three issues here. First, Terry did not get the reports to you on time. Second, you brought this to his attention. And, third, he became aggressive and told you to mind your own business."

The skill of reflective summary is one of the more critical and powerful in the leader's arsenal for three reasons: It demonstrates engaged listening; it provides an opportunity for correction and clarification on certain points, and it moves forward, which is especially important when the speaker is rambling or pursuing unrelated tangents.

Selective silence and reflective summary are generally followed by the final piece of this triad, "reflective meaning." Reflective meaning allows you touch on the understory. It is your perception of the emotion and meaning that comes through as you have listened to the other party. Reflective meaning is interpretive, but it is not judgmental, and it is not elaborative. You are reflecting the emotion and meaning that seem to be part of the message that you have just heard. For example, "If I have heard you correctly, the situation with Terry has left you frustrated and angry. You feel that he has treated you in a disrespectful manner that simply cannot be tolerated here."

A caveat is needed at this point. Many of us tend to either affirm or counter the reflective meaning we have just noted. In other words, we take an additional evaluative step. For example, "You should be mad; I'd be mad, too." Or, "Terry is a good person. He's just under a lot of pressure right now." Such evaluative commentary is best left for subsequent dialogue (which we will discuss shortly) or when the other party offers you a point of entry by requesting your opinion.

There is a final theme, a consideration that can change the entire nature of the listening exchange. It has to do with pace. As busy, intense, quick studies, with a plate full of issues, you work in contexts where the pace of interactions is ramped up. Consequently, it will come as no surprise that one of our most frequent encouragements to physician leaders desiring to enhance the skill of engaged listening is quite simple: Slow the pace of interaction. Speak a bit more slowly. Allow a bit more of an interlude between the back-and-forth handoffs that characterize all interpersonal exchanges. Difficult as it can be, slowing the pace of exchange portrays a tone that encourages the other party to speak more while signaling your desire to reflect more.

Expansive Questioning and Humble Inquiry

We all understand the difference between closed questions (requiring brief, limited and often single-phrase responses) and open-ended questions (that require deeper explanations). Certainly there are times and places where closed questions are necessary and expedient. "Is she stable?" "Is your blood pressure normally this high?" "Has this product failed before?"

Open-ended questions, while taking additional time, allow others more range in their replies and hopefully provide us with more data and greater understanding. "What difficulties are the nurses having with the new policy?" "How will this strategy affect our overall costs?" Expansive questioning relies heavily on open-ended questions. However, there is more.

Edgar Schein is a giant in the organizational development field. His research and writing have shaped our thinking in many areas. For example, his studies of organizational culture have provided original, cutting-edge insights and perspectives on what culture means and why it is so important. Schein's most recent work is a thoughtful and deeply personal book, *Humble Inquiry*. While exploring the depths of inquiry and helping us reframe our interpersonal approaches, the book is, in many ways, an homage to his wife, Mary. Consider the scenario described below.

"When my wife Mary had her first bout of breast cancer in her 50s, we were sent to an oncologist who immediately conveyed to her an interest

in her total personality and life situation through body language (intense attention and eye contact), through taking lots of time with questions, and always responding sympathetically. ...He asked her several general and personal questions before zeroing in on the medically related issues. My wife felt respected as a total human being and therefore felt more open to voicing her concerns about treatment. ...What was striking was his questioning about our other life priorities, which made Mary feel that she could trust him totally."[18]

"Humble inquiry is the fine art of drawing someone out, of asking questions to which you do not already know the answers, of building a relationship based on curiosity and interest in the other person," Schein said. [19] As such, humble inquiry is far more than mere questioning. By assuming an attitude of curiosity and interest toward another person, it resonates with a "desire to build a relationship" with that person.[20] Schein's points could hardly be more relevant or timely.

Schein offers a twist — what may be for some a rather novel way to think about and approach interpersonal exchanges. Understandably, your clinical background and experiences may have fostered an "informational" rather than "relational" approach to questioning. This does not suggest that you are insensitive. Nor does it suggest that you eschew relationships. Rather, the informational approach views questioning as an exchange or transaction to secure key information to make a more informed decision. Accordingly, immediacy and speed of exchange are keys. Make no mistake, you face many contexts (often driven by time constraints) when informational questioning is essential and completely appropriate.

What we sometimes miss is that every question, even those with purely informational intentions, creates relational impact. Additionally, as noted earlier, we tend to be problem solvers rather than people who use nuanced probes of inquiry. Schein's advice is direct and clear: "We must become better at asking and do less telling in a culture that overvalues telling."[21]

This change is not simple and often requires breaking well-entrenched assumptions and habits. The message has particular meaning for physician leaders. The assertions may drive to the heart of the physician worldview where the common tendency is to "value task accomplishment over relationship building and (where we) either are not aware of this cultural bias or, worse, don't care and don't want to be bothered with it."[22]

There is a deeper dynamic at play. As stated earlier, in many clinical contexts, informational inquiry is what we desire. For example, a physician may ask the attending nurse for an update on a problematic patient's night under observation in the hospital. The physician seeks information — data that will enable an accurate assessment and determination of the next course of action. Expansive inquiry takes the next step, as the physician asks the nurse, "Is there anything you observed that we need to consider here? Anything that might be important to consider for our next steps?" This approach is expansive from an informational point of view because it seeks input and perspective that is unavailable elsewhere. This approach is expansive from a relational point of view because it signals to the nurse that he or she is a significant part of the team whose input is both sought and desired.

When we move from clinical to administrative activities, the nature of expansive inquiry becomes even more important. Here, you grapple with situations where clarity is clouded and facts are limited. Further, even the facts you have are open to broad and at times opposing interpretations.

While we are cautious of formulaic designations when dealing with bright people, we believe that expansive questioning and inquiry work best when three themes are considered and used.

Similar to what we discussed with engaged listening, expansive questioning begins with assuming and projecting a "genuine interest" in the other party. That includes a genuine interest in what they have to say, as well as the logic and emotion behind the statements that are being uttered. Next, we should "minimize our preconceptions" about the other party. We will say more about this shortly, as we discuss dialogue.

Finally, we must "probe for understanding" by using open, exploratory questions. It is important to realize that thoughtful and respectful probes for understanding are predicated on the establishment of a tone of genuine interest and a willingness to engage other parties with a tone of inquiry that is void of preconceptions and assumptions of intent. Without these elements in place, others are likely to see probing questions as harsh, invasive, critical or, as a team member once shared, "just digging and searching to show me where I am wrong."

Probing and exploratory questions are generally denoted by "why" and "how." While useful and encouraged, other probing styles can be more meaningful and enhancing. Here, we encourage you to listen for and probe when the other party offers you a "natural opening." For example, "As I listened to you describe our experiences with that supplier; you noted that there have been a couple of glitches in the past. Could you tell us more about those?" Or, "You said your experiences with Jenny have mostly been positive. Would it be useful for me to understand the exceptions, and if so, what are they?" One of our favorite probes is the simple phrase "Help me understand." "Help me understand more about your relationship with Jenny."

As noted earlier, the decision to use probing and exploratory questions takes time. There will be some side roads, and you will probably have to help the other party stay focused by returning to the issues at hand. We encourage a direct and respectful approach. Yet always be cognizant that an apparent side track may be revelatory, suggesting another probe that mines the true depth of the issue at hand.

Conflicting Messages

Extensive research into the ways we communicate — linguistically, pa-ra-linguistically (accompanying sounds that connote emotion and meaning) and nonverbally — underscores what we have learned through experience. Meaning is derived from all sources, but the truth of one's words can be undermined by conflicting actions that fall outside the realm of basic linguistic exchanges. Common here is the classic double-bind message, where we verbally send one message and simultaneously send another (often nonverbally) that conflicts with or refutes the initial message. For example, consider the leader who contends that he wants people to "feel free to share what's on your mind," but begins to fidget and glance at his phone once meaningful conversation unfolds.

Not surprisingly, the nonverbal message generally overpowers the verbal one, as people infer that the nonverbal message is more indicative of the leader's true intention and motive. In fact, researchers have suggested that 65 to 70 percent of our emotional interpretations may be derived from nonverbal sources.[23] A dismissive roll of the eyes, a sarcastic "humph" (a paralinguistic), or an exasperated shrug of the shoulders can undermine most verbal messages. And there is an additional factor. Double-binds are likely to be perceived as disrespectful and diminishing, destroying interpersonal trust and increasing hesitancy to engage in dialogue.

A simple example that we have probably all experienced drives home the point. At a staff meeting we attended, the leader asked for feedback, heralding the value of the staff's views. One of the nurses spoke up and offered some thoughts on a potential work-flow bottleneck. As the nurse spoke (a succinct 15- or 20-second statement), the physician glanced at his watch not once but twice — a behavior that all observed. Not surprisingly, there were no additional comments.

The Dynamics of Dialogue

The ability to lead others through thoughtful, respectful and revelatory dialogue is one the most important skills of contemporary leadership. In simplest terms, dialogue is a conversation — a word that should not be dismissed or minimized by its apparent simplicity. In a two-year study of organizational communication, Boris Groysberg and Michael Slind interviewed professionals from more than 100 companies. Among their findings, "Smart leaders today ... engage employees in a way that resembles an ordinary person-to-person conversation more than it does a series of commands from on high."[24]

As a conversation, dialogue occurs within a complex context, laden with emotional undertones and diverse needs. In short, every party enters the dialogue with unique needs and a sense of meaning. As an interactive exchange, dialogue strives to deepen collective understanding and insight, resulting in enhanced, collaborative decisions and actions. True dialogue results in "the free flow of meaning between two or more people," thereby expanding the "pool of shared meaning."[25] When done correctly, dialogue leads to improved trust, better decisions and deeper levels of buy-in.[26]

As pragmatists, we recognize that every situation and decision does not require dialogue. Indeed, some situations beg for leaders to make unilateral calls. In such situations, involving others leads to confusion, undermines credibility and wastes time. Generally, if the leader possesses all the information needed to make a decision, is assured that others' acceptance or buy-in will be present and is facing the pressure of time, a unilateral decision is justified.[27] However, even these guidelines are often clouded by subtleties that hamper our capacity to check off each requirement with reasonable certainty.

Leaders face a range of decisions that are quite nuanced. Procedural clarity that may drive action in certain clinical settings rarely exists as you discuss strategic direction with disparate stakeholders. Financial metrics, while seemingly definitive, are open to varied interpretations and are generally skewed by self-interests. Human resource decisions are even more problematic. Policy, legality, motivational impact and the creation of implied precedent must all be considered.

Divergent views — all with some degree of merit — exist. Parties have their own frames of reference, coupled with idiosyncratic styles of expression. Deep emotions are involved, prompting people to be willing to dig in and fight rather than dispassionately accept the directions of others.

In many ways, your leadership is defined and your reputation is built by how you respond and finesse these situations. As decision complexity increases and divergence of views broadens, dialogue becomes an important method of response.

Disparate Needs and Varied Agendas

Again, let's think of dialogue as a conversation or discussion among invested parties who come together to reach a collective decision. As in any exchange, each participating party has special needs and unique personal agendas. Sometimes those needs and agendas mesh. At other times, they clash, and the ensuing discussion derails as disparate needs and varied agendas are pursued. And, like it or not, personal agendas may trump collective goals, threatening a condition of suboptimization, where one unit or department gains while all others lose. This is the unspoken behavioral backdrop that is present in every serious discussion.

Even more problematic is the elusive demon of the "hidden agenda." Here, one or more parties positions and plots while others are trying to figure out what the understory really is. The apparent logic is fairly uncomplicated. Some participants believe that if they openly share their needs, their political hand will be tipped, leverage will be lost and their pet agendas will remain largely unrealized. Make no mistake, the hidden agenda creates a destructive scenario. It undermines good decisions and it destroys trust. The guarded tone that emerges within a team or group drains psychological energy and wastes time.[28]

Consider the insidious nature of the hidden agenda as it was expressed by one member of a multi-department team describing the behavior of another member.

> *"Every statement he makes is angling toward some eventual outcome that he wants. It's always an outcome that benefits him and his unit. So I can never take his comments at face value. I'm always trying to figure out what's going on. Why is he saying this? And how am I going to get screwed in the process?"*

Dialogue, by its very nature, attempts to reduce the haunting presence of the hidden agenda.

The Keys to Successful Dialogue

We realize that dialogue, much like trust, is a concept that is readily espoused and too infrequently achieved. The elusive nature of true dialogue arises from the tenuous nature of a set of undergirding assumptions that are difficult to embrace in practice. Six assumptions (and resulting behaviors) are key and should be met for dialogue to flourish and realize its full potential. These assumptions are: all parties must have opportunities to contribute and add their meaning to the discussion; all parties must be interested in listening to one another; differing points of view and perspectives must be valued and respected; parties must be willing to suspend their preconceived beliefs and judgments; all parties must be willing to reflect on and actively consider perspectives that differ from their own, and parties must be open and willing to be changed through the interactive and reflective process.[29]

These key assumptions provide the essential framework. However, in many ways, they are aspirational assumptions — ideals that are regularly disrupted and violated by the vagaries of real people working in competitive and politically charged contexts. Accordingly, it is the leader's responsibility to facilitate and create an environment of meaningful dialogue.

To do so, you must truly believe in the value of dialogue. You must believe, as experts assert, that dialogue mobilizes our collective talent.[30] Next, we encourage you to share the six assumptions as new teams begin their work

— asserting that these assumptions create the attitudinal and behavioral tone for successful collaboration. And, as leaders, you will need to intervene periodically to help ensure that members are adhering to the fundamentals. Here, rather than chastising undesired behavior, you model appropriate behavior. For example, "Let's return to Bob's point. I'm not sure we probed the depths of his contribution."

Blockers

One way to improve dialogue is to recognize and address some of the common reasons it goes off course. These so-called blockers of dialogue exist in nearly every exchange. We will explore three common tendencies and biases that demand attention.

The first blocker is the interpersonal dynamic known as "groupthink."[31] More than 50 years ago, Yale psychologist Irving Janis and his colleagues conducted a series of investigations to try to understand why very bright groups of people can come together, engage in dialogue and yet make unbelievably clumsy decisions. Janis' work was prompted by the 1961 Bay of Pigs fiasco during the presidency of John Kennedy. Given the collective talent of Kennedy's Cabinet — arguably one of the more intellectually elite in history — how could they make such flawed and seemingly obvious mistakes, including the decision to invade Cuba?

What Janis found has become a fundamental caveat in group dynamics. It seems that the Cabinet members, as individuals, had strong reservations about the emerging mission, but the group had become so strong and cohesive that individuals were unwilling to dissent or "rock the boat." The group, collectively, displayed a "norm to conform" that Janis labeled "groupthink." In Janis' words, groupthink is "a mode of thinking that people engage in when they are deeply involved in a cohesive in-group, when the members' strivings for unanimity override their motivation to realistically appraise alternative courses of action."[32] In strongly supportive and cohesive groups, consensus becomes more important than tough queries of pending risks and possible flaws.

Importantly, as groups become more cohesive, the tendency toward groupthink increases — a damning two-edged sword. On one hand, we desire collaboration and cohesiveness. On the other hand, consensus can deter critical evaluation. In the process, the impact of dialogue falls short because of an unwillingness to express and consider contrarian views.

Leadership becomes paramount. We must be alert to signs of groupthink. For example, when complex decisions receive strong initial support from all parties, red flags should be flashing in your mind. You may need to encourage dissenting views. You may need to make sure risks are debated and assessed. You may need to legitimize the devil's advocate role as a cautionary dynamic that becomes part of the conversation.

Most important, you should be acutely aware of individual and group tactics aimed at squelching dissenting views. Often these attempts are subtle and emotionally based, as simple as, "Gee, Joe, everyone else seems to be onboard." Or the tactics can be more aggressive — "Joe, at this rate, we'll be never get this project completed." The ultimate minimizing tactic is to take a quick vote, virtually assuring that the dissenter's views will be dismissed.

In all cases, these tactics depart from logical analysis in favor of deflection and speedy agreement. The leader walks a fine line. You must plumb the dissenting arguments for clarity, understanding and value, but you must also forward the action.

Our preference is for group members to articulate the concerns of dissenters, validate those concerns and affirm their willingness to accept the risks of disagreeing with the dissenters and moving on. As the leader, you may need to play the role of ensuring that these steps have been taken. For example:

> *"OK, we understand that Joe is concerned that this decision could place additional burdens on our emergency department. We have talked through and assessed the risks involved. Joe has helped us understand that our communication with the ED staff needs to occur early in the process. We all agree. It also seems that we are willing to accept the risks Joe has mentioned because of the overall value of the project. So let's move on."*

Leadership sincerity and authenticity are important here. Dissenting opinions need to be considered; at times they provide awareness of issues that must be addressed, yet they cannot derail the overall decision-making process. Above all, the framing above is respectful of Joe and helps assure that important, albeit divergent, perspectives are fully considered.

Our second blocker is a behavioral theme known as the "commitment bias."[33] The commitment bias suggests that team members enter the dialogue discussion having already studied the issues and established deep perspectives and impressions of actions that are needed. In short, members arrive with some degree of commitment to a course of action. Logically, the more fully one has studied an issue, had similar experiences and feels that his expertise extends to the issue at hand, the deeper the level of commitment. The presence of the commitment bias assures that we do not think in fresh and open ways. Rather, we tend to be closely wed to our well-studied and strongly felt preconceived perspectives. Parties are locked in an internal reasoning process that suggests "Why should I move from my well-reasoned commitments?" To some extent, we all fall prey to the trap of the commitment bias.

Knowing this, what do we do? First, it is important to hear all perspectives before anyone engages in a deep and protracted lobbying effort. The wonderful adage that "everyone speaks once before anyone speaks twice" can be a tone changer.[34] Second, it is important to make sure that divergent, even seemingly offbeat perspectives are provided a fair hearing and reasoned consideration. Third, ask questions of those holding differing perspectives. Here, the path of humble inquiry makes sense. Your questions, at least initially, should not target elements of disagreement but should seek to deepen understanding and add clarity. We encourage the use of "help me understand" questions.

As process observers during a partner meeting of physicians in a clinical practice, we saw this play out. One partner, Steve, expressed a strongly felt view that dissented from the majority. Another partner, Dave, with a tone of intellectual dismissal, turned to Steve and commented, "That just doesn't make any sense." As expected, Steve's counter-response was defensive and strongly assertive. Another partner, Greg, quickly intervened, turned toward Steve and asked the humble inquiry questions. "Steve, I know you feel strongly about Option B. Will you help me understand why? What are you seeing that I may be missing?"

There is a pragmatic point to Greg's inquiry. The team, in reality, may be missing something. More deeply, two important behavioral facets are underscored by Greg's inquiry — acknowledgement and legitimacy. Acknowledgement and legitimacy are not agreement. Rather, they represent a fundamental understanding that talented people can hold differing views. Steve had uncovered a complexity in the majority opinion that had not been fully explored. Once the team acknowledged this issue and discussed its impact, Steve was satisfied. "OK, I'm convinced this is not as big a deal as I thought it was. I'm OK with Option A."

With a bias for transparency, we must finish this story. As you have probably assumed, Steve's foray added an additional 15 minutes to the discussion. However, it is also true that an important and previously unrealized risk was discussed and subsequently dismissed, and a key team player was onboard and fully supportive of the final decision. We would like to report that all partners recognized and appreciated the long-term impact of Greg's intervention, but behaviors are deeply ingrained and change slowly. Leaving the conference room, Dave glanced at me, flipped his head toward Steve, and softly commented, "I knew he was wrong!"

Next, let's consider a final blocker — the "power bias." The power bias is a natural factor present in all interpersonal exchanges. In short, this bias occurs because some individuals (usually by virtue of expertise, reputation or position) are accorded higher status than others in an exchange. As such, the views of these power elite are accorded higher levels of consideration and impact than their less powerful counterparts. (It is easy to assert that during dialogue, all parties are extended equal power. But it simply is not true, and it is impossible to enact, especially when issues become heated and individual perspectives are deeply felt.) As we have noted repeatedly, when working in cross-disciplinary teams, physicians (usually by virtue of your specialized expertise and social status) carry differential power.

Some individuals use their power as a conscious lever, wielded selectively to secure agreement and dissuade dissent on certain issues. Others are less aware of the sway they carry because team members defer to them more naturally and subtly out of respect for their expertise or hierarchical level. Interestingly, while purity of motive may differ, impact does not. Careful, involved and unbiased discussion is threatened.

Again, it is the leader's responsibility to minimize the coercive nature of these power differentials. The rules and guidelines we have noted for other biases certainly can be used here.

Concluding Thoughts: The Need for Action

This chapter has championed three tone-setting themes: engaged listening, expansive questioning and dialogue. These themes help establish a safe and collaborative environment where the best ideas can surface and be considered. We have argued, directly and by implication, that doing so enhances employee commitment and leads to better decisions. Now we face the reality of execution — the need to move beyond dialogue — the need to take action.

In Chapter 2, we made the case for leader decisiveness. We recognized that leaders must step forward, make tough decisions and act, often in the midst of uncertainty and incomplete information. Dialogue, by expanding meaning and opening discussions to varied (and at times hidden) perspectives, offers the hope of reducing uncertainty and bridging informational gaps.

In addition, dialogue is a critical tool of persuasion. Since those affected by decisions have been offered voice and respectful inquiry, they have a clearer view of why decisions are being made. Further, as active participants in the process of discussion, they feel a sense of ownership and are more likely to accept and support final decisions, even if those decisions did not take the exact course that they desired.

In his outstanding work on influence, Robert Cialdini addresses the psychology of persuasion. In one of our favorite sections, Cialdini leads us into the dichotomous nature of interpersonal exchanges — exchanges that must be deciphered and coalesced into action.

> *"Very often in making a decision about someone or something, we don't use all the relevant available information; we use, instead, only a single, highly representative piece of the total. And an isolated piece of information, even though it normally counsels us correctly, can lead us to clearly stupid mistakes. ...At the same time (there is) a complicating companion theme. ...Despite the susceptibility to stupid decisions that accompanies a reliance on a single feature of the available data, the pace of modern life demands that we frequently use this shortcut."*[35]

Leaders from all professions battle the demon of time. Yet none may be more sensitive to the crushing limits of time as those engaged in clinical activities. In some cases, speed of decisions is essential to patient welfare. In other cases, systemic demands for efficiency limit exchanges. Questions are asked to fill in the pieces to permit a confident course of action — actions with gauged and acceptable outcome probabilities. The risk of hesitation and indecisiveness is costly, and your training and experience have helped you engage in cognitive assessments to mitigate those risks. To a large part, you have traversed the chasm that Cialdini described by being smart enough to ask the right questions.

In short, there are times, as a leader, when you must step up and take action. Despite the value of bringing the involved parties together and engaging in the impactful processes discussed in this chapter, you simply cannot. Immediacy of action is needed and a unilateral decision is warranted. Largely, we believe that others accept the need for decisiveness because of situational realities. Importantly, they will accept your actions because of the consistent tone of engagement and dialogue that is your normal and predominant style of interaction.

---

1. Frese, M.; Beimel, S.; & Schoenborn, S. (2003). Action training for charismatic leadership: Two evaluations of studies of a commercial training module on inspirational communication of a vision. *Personnel Psychology*, 56(3), 671-697. Kirkpatrick, S.A. & Locke, E.A. (1996). Direct and indirect effects of three core charismatic leadership components on performance and attitudes. *Journal of Applied Psychology*, 81, 36-51. Towler, A.J. (2003). Effects of charismatic influence training on attitudes, behavior, and performance. *Personnel Psychology*, 56(2), 363-381.

2. Harrell, T.W. & Harrell, M.S. (1984). *Stanford MBA careers: A 20-year longitudinal study.* Graduate School Business Research Paper, No. 723. Stanford, CA.

3. McKenna, M.K.; Gartland, M.P.; & Pugno, P.A. (20004). Development of physician leadership competencies: Perceptions of physician leaders, physician educators and medical students. *Journal of Health Administration Education, 21*(3), 343-354.

4. Bawany, S. (2014). Great leaders are good communicators. *Leadership Excellence,* 31.

5. Bambacus, M. & Patrickson, M. (2008). Interpersonal communication skills that enhance organizational commitment. *Journal of Communication Management,* 12(1), 51-72.

6. Nellermoe, D.A.; Weirich, T.R.; & Reinstein, A. (1999). Using practitioners' viewpoints to improve accounting students' communication skills. *Business Communication Quarterly,* 62(2), 41-60.

7. Porter, M.E. & Nohria, N. (2010). What is leadership: The CEO's role in large complex organizations. In Nohria, N. & Khuruna, R. (eds.), *Handbook of Leadership Theory and Practice.* Boston: Harvard Business Press.

8. Reported in, Adler, R.B.; Rosenfeld, L.B.; & Proctor II, R.F. (2013). *Interplay: The process of interpersonal communication.* New York: Oxford University Press.

9. Calloway-Thomas, C.; Cooper, P.; & Blake, C. (1999). *Interpersonal communication: Roots and routes.* Upper Saddle River, NJ: Pearson.

10. Stoner, C.R. & Stoner, J.S. (2013). *Building leaders: Paving the path for emerging leaders.* New York: Routledge.

11. Ibid.

12. Duck, J.D. (1998). Managing change: The art of balancing. *Harvard Business Review, 71*(6), 109-118.

13. Covey, S.R. (1989). *The 7 Habits of Highly Successful People: Powerful lessons in personal change.* New York: Fireside.

14. Stoner, C.R. & Stoner, J.S. (2014). How can we make this work: Understanding and responding to working parents of children with autism. *Business Horizons, 57*(1), 85-95.

15. Langer, E. (1990). *Mindfulness.* Reading, MA: Addison-Wesley.

16. Cloke, K. & Goldsmith, J. (2011). *Resolving Conflicts at Work: Ten strategies for everyone on the job.* San Francisco: Jossey-Bass.

17. Goleman, D. *Social Intelligence: The revolutionary new science of human relationship.* New York: Bantam Books, p. 86.

18. Schein, E.H. (2013). *Humble Inquiry: The gentle art of asking instead of telling.* San Francisco: Berrett-Koehler, pp. 34-35.

19. Ibid.

20. Ibid., p. 19.

21. Ibid., p. 3.

22. Ibid., p. 55.

23. Birdwhistell, R.L. (1970). *Kinesics and context.* Philadelphia: University of Pennsylvania Press. Mehrabian, A. (1972). *Nonverbal communication.* Chicago: Aldine-Atherton.

24. Groysberg, B. & Slind, M. (2012). Leadership is a conversation: How to improve employee engagement and alignment in today's flatter, more networked organizations. *Harvard Business Review,* June, 76-84, p. 78.

25. Patterson, K.; Grenny, J.; McMillan, R.; & Switzler, A. (2002). *Crucial Conversations: Tools for talking when the stakes are high.* New York: McGraw-Hill, pp. 20-21.

26. Hardy, C.; Lawrence, T.B.; & Grant, D. (2005). Discourse and collaboration: The role of conversations and collective identity. *Academy of Management Review,* 30, 58-77.

27. Vroom, V.H. & Jago, A.G. (1988). *The New Leadership: Managing participation in organizations.* Englewood Cliffs, NJ: Prentice-Hall.

28. An interesting perspective here is offered by Covey. Covey, S.M.R.

29. Raelin, J. (2012). The manager as facilitator of dialogue. *Organization,* 20(6), 818-839. Bohm, D. (1996). *On Dialogue.* London: Routledge.

30. Raelin, J. (2003). *Creating Leaderful Organizations: How to bring out leadership in everyone.* San Francisco: Berrett-Koehler.

31. Janis, I.L. (1972). *Victims of Groupthink: A psychological study of foreign policy decisions and fiascoes.* Boston: Houghton-Mifflin. Essser, J.K. (1998). Alive and well after 25 years: A review of groupthink research. *Organizational Behavior and Human Decision Processes, 73*(2-3), 116-141.

32. Janis, I.L. (1982). *Victims of Groupthink* (2nd ed.). Boston: Houghton-Mifflin, p. 9.

33. Staw, B.M. (1976). Knee deep in the big muddy: A study of escalating commitment to a chosen course of action. *Organizational Behavior and Human Performance,* 16(1), 27-44.

34. Brafman, O. & Brafman, R. (2008). *Sway: The irresistible pull of irrational behavior.* New York: Doubleday.

35. Cialdini, R.B. (2007). Influence: the Psychology of Persuasion. New York: Harper., p. 274.

5

Teamwork: The Foundations
of Collective Synergy

....

IN THE DOCUMENTARY *THE WAITING ROOM*, THE CHAOS OF AN EMER-
gency room is captured on film. The movie focuses on the doctors, nurses, administrative staff, EMTs and hospital security officers at a public hospital as they work to serve their patients. The EMTs rush into the emergency room with a patient on a gurney who has suffered a gunshot wound to the head. The nurses and doctors quickly surround the patient. Doctors spring into action, assessing the situation and giving orders to nurses with short, concise statements. Nurses bustle around, acting on the doctor's orders. It is a scene of a medical team in action.

In today's workplace, teams are the means of doing business. However, when we ask people across organizational levels if they like working in teams, the answer is not always positive. Consider a recent study that polled more than 1,000 Americans. Although 95 percent of the respondents found value in teamwork, nearly 75 percent of the respondents preferred not to work in teams.[1]

Many saw potential value in teamwork, including the opportunity to bring together diverse resources to accomplish goals that would be unattainable with the resources of one individual. At the same time, respondents viewed teamwork as a deterrent to progress. Unreliable team members were a constant source of frustration and stress. Team members with different paces of work were viewed as an annoyance. And, of course, fears of carrying others' responsibilities — picking up the slack for those less talented and less motivated — was always a concern.

As physicians, you know the benefit of having a well-functioning and productive team. You have the clarity to realize that your job would be more difficult, if not impossible, without team-focused support from nurses, administrative staff and support personnel. In part, this awareness arises because of the specialized skills that each team participant brings to the table.

Often the team works toward an integrated goal with clear responsibilities and handoffs that are smooth and efficient. Consider a family practice. Here, the family practitioner (FP) knows that a patient needs a certain drug and sets the team interplay in motion. The FP asks the nurse to give the injection and moves on to the next patient. The nurse gives the injection and then is on to take the next set of orders from the doctor. The administrative staff takes care of the financial transaction with the patient, files the insurance claims and documents the patient's visit. No doubt a single physician could handle all of these activities, but only if the volume rate was nearly zero. With a well-functioning team in place, the physician can see more patients and concentrate on providing each with the best medical treatment.

Yet teams and the assumptions of collaborative problem solving can be taxing for physicians who are trained to be fiercely independent. To all of this we must add an unfortunate reality. Most of us have worked in a dysfunctional team setting. Perhaps we have members of our team who are not as talented as their role requires. Perhaps we have team members we simply do not like. Perhaps we are working with individuals who possess different overarching goals than our own.

Even when formed with the best intentions and talent and working toward a mutually accepted goal, teams often do not perform at optimal levels. The performance potential of teams is considerable, yet that potential is realized only with careful attention to team leadership and overall team dynamics. These are the dominant themes that will be addressed throughout this chapter.

A Sense of Teams

At the most basic level, a team can be described as "interdependent collections of individuals who share responsibility for specific outcomes."[2] Probing more deeply, Jon Katzenbach and Douglas Smith offered a longer but insightful definition of a team: "A *small number of people* with *complementary skills* who are committed to a *common purpose, performance goals* and *working approach,* for which they hold themselves *mutually accountable.*"[3] The power of the definition resides in the six "team basics" (highlighted in italics) that are essential for high-performing teams.

We add another dimension to the definitional mix. Often, people are grouped together, labeled as a team and encouraged to work together. In some cases, these remain pseudo-teams at best and they exhibit few if any of the defining characteristics set forth above. At times, we have little more than a collection of individuals, each pursuing individual interests. For a team to have performance impact, its members must be willing to subjugate self-interests at key decision-making junctures. Unless this act of escalating team over self occurs, teams exist in name only.

Consider a common example. A nine-person, cross-functional team was established to consider reorganization of one area of a regional hospital. The team was composed of an array of talent with representative clinicians, as well as those from financial and strategic administrative areas. During brainstorming in the early months, the team functioned openly and efficiently. Then, a day of reckoning was at hand. Finally forced to make some tough decisions that would significantly change the way certain areas operated, the demon of turf protection reared its head. With few exceptions, the members were open to change in any area except their own. One member even boldly challenged his peers: "You can change anything else, but I'll tell you one area (his area) that will not change."

Teams are designed to create synergy — to reach the "synergistic advantage." Working with others we hope to accomplish more and make better decisions than we could as individuals. We gain synergistic advantages in three ways. First, and most obvious, we bring together individuals whose backgrounds, experiences, talents and perspectives represent diverse arenas. As such, this "diversity effect" enriches the pool of inputs and ideas, injecting opportunities for creativity and forward-thinking decisions. Such diversity also helps us avoid pitfalls by broadening our understanding of the complexity of the situations we face.

Second, synergy rests on an "expansive effect." As team members openly share and engage others in discussion, we begin to see new ways to combine ideas, link strategies and embrace fresh actions that are truly unique contributions garnered from a variety of sources.

Third, synergy rests on the concept of social facilitation.[4] By working with others, at least in some cases, people can feel pushed to add extra effort. They can even feel a deeper sense of accountability because others are aware of their comments and actions. As such, we may be able to experience deeper levels of commitment and higher levels of performance, presumably because of the presence of others and the desire to not let teammates down.

Of course, many of you have experienced a different team dynamic — a negative synergy. For example, at times, team members can slough off and fail to pull their weight, often assuming that someone else on the team (usually hard-driving perfectionists) will pick up the slack and make sure that both quality and timeliness of outcomes are achieved. This phenomenon, known as social loafing or free-riding, diminishes team impact and morale.[5]

In general, negative synergy stems from issues of team size, lack of clarity regarding purpose and direction and debilitating interpersonal exchanges. Quite notably, negative synergy can also arise when strong, dominant members push teams in errant directions, often because other team members shut down rather than offer opposition.

In many ways, your role as both team leader and team member is to facilitate an interactional framework for enabling synergistic advantages while limiting negative synergy. We will discuss and offer thoughts on how to reach these desired outcomes in the following pages. In these discussions, we explore two main topics: how to build a team and how to lead a team by managing team processes. In the next section, we focus on providing you with a frame of reference for teamwork. Then, basic guidelines for building a team will be considered. Finally, the bulk of the chapter will focus on the leader actions to ensure maximum long-term performance.

The Stages of Team Formation

To grasp the dynamics of teams more fully, consider the five stages of group (or team) formation.[6] The first stage — "forming" — involves the designation and assembly of new team members. During this stage, conversations are generally polite and superficial. Team values as well as acceptable and unacceptable behaviors are being clarified at this stage. The second stage — "storming" — involves conflict as team members challenge one another regarding both direction and leadership. Importantly, this conflict leads to deeper understanding and acceptance of the goals of the group, the roles that each team member will play, and the early emergence of performance norms.

The storming stage is a necessary process so that groups can reach the third stage — "norming." In this stage, groups become uniform in their understanding of who they are, what they are to do and how they will do it. Team leadership emerges and is legitimized during this stage. Once this stage is completed, groups progress to the "performing" stage. As goals are reached and closure is at hand, the team experiences the "adjourning" stage.

As a leader, it's important to note the natural progression of these stages and the natural and important stage of conflict. Both the pace and the conflict are uncomfortable for most leaders, who wish to lead an efficient and functional team. During the storming stage, however, the team often appears to be dysfunctional. As a leader, you must embrace some degree of friction in order for the team to develop shared norms. The chapter on conflict in this book will help with that process, but the important point right now is to exhibit patience during this stage. Embrace it; work through it with the goal of setting high performance work norms; maintain the highest levels of interpersonal respect, even in the face of disagreement, and the effort will pay dividends in the long run.

How to Build a Team

There is a difference between a work group and a team. In general, work groups are individuals who are working toward a common goal, and they do so by completing individual tasks and then aggregating their efforts. Conversely, teams are individuals who are working toward a common goal that have higher elements of coordination and experience synergistic advantages. In some ways, teams are work groups that perform at a high level by not only using the diverse set of resources each team member brings to the team, but also by having higher-quality interactions. As a leader, you are responsible for shaping your work groups into high-performing work teams. Luckily, there is an abundance of literature and research about this key leadership challenge.

More than 30 years ago, J.R. Hackman first proposed his input-process-outcome model for understanding the design and management of teams.[7] Since then, many researchers have examined his model and added to it. With an admission of selectivity, we will review some of the more salient aspects of this research and consider some foundational best practices.

Team Size

One important consideration that must be addressed, even at this early juncture, has to do with team size. Experts recognize that while a team must have representational dynamics that are consistent with its purpose, the numbers simply cannot become too large.

We have all seen the membership roster bulge, often with poor outcomes. As team membership grows, we experience a country club effect, where side roads of socialization pull the team off task. At other times, the size becomes so large that cliques and factions fracture the direction and intensity of the team's work. For years, researchers have searched for the right number — cognizant that the answer depends largely on the context, the range of talent and the task.

Conventional wisdom notes that teams should be composed of 5-7, 7-9 or 9-12 individuals.[8] These are rough rules of thumb, however. As teams become larger, coordination becomes more difficult.[9] Based on the research, it seems best to make teams as small as possible while meeting your representational needs. This will limit the opportunities for social loafing by allowing the team members to feel more task identity. Jon Katzenbach and Douglas Smith suggest that the number generally should be fewer than 12.[10] Another good rule here is to attempt to have odd numbers in the group to avoid an indecisive split at key decision-making junctures.

Intact or Rotating Teams

One of the basic elements that has been empirically demonstrated time and again is that long-standing, or intact, teams outperform temporary, or rotating, teams. This may seem counterintuitive, in that there is a perception that long-standing teams suffer from too much familiarity and eventual groupthink (see the previous chapter). Yet the positive potential of intact teams seems compelling.

First, the learning curve advantages of familiarity seem to trump the possible disadvantages. For example, in a massive study of more than 1,000 development projects conducted through a software services company, researchers found that a 50 percent increase in team familiarity correlated with a 19 percent reduction in defects, a 30 percent decrease in budget deviations and a 10 percent improvement in performance. The authors boldly noted that "familiarity helps team members share information and communicate effectively, (and) it makes them more likely to integrate knowledge and come up with a coherent, innovative solution."[11] Similar findings have been found in an array of teams, including surgical teams.[12]

In short, intact teams seem to experience higher degrees of coordination, better use of specialized skills and more effective communication processes.[13] Of course, we must be ever diligent. There is no doubt that teams can be together too long.

Although long-standing teams have progressed through key developmental and learning phases, all teams have to start somewhere. At times, as a leader, you have the opportunity to start from scratch to design your team. By properly designing a team, you are able to craft a better probability of team success.

Clarity and Acceptance: Distal Goals

As with most efforts, teams will flounder without both a clear understanding and member acceptance of the central purpose. In turn, this central purpose should be translated into the team's overall, or distal, goal.

In fact, the determination of the team's distal goal is the initial step for building a team. This sounds rather elementary, but there is a deeper issue. As a leader, you need to recognize the difference between being a clinical physician in a team and being a physician leader at the helm of the team. The goals that you are pursuing as a team leader cannot be self-serving but must be focused toward the greater good of the followers and/or the organization.

As a leader, you must think about the team goals in their entirety, taking into account systems thinking and considering all stakeholders. Systems thinking attempts to view all pieces as interlocking "mini" systems that aggregate to a greater system. As a leader, you should be able to look at the organization and the competitive environment and determine how your team's part plays into the larger system and understand how changes in other parts of the system will affect your team. Also, leaders need to consider all the relevant stakeholders. The goal is for your team's actions to affect other teams and individuals so that value is added to the organization. Your orientation should be geared toward the question "what is the goal of the team and how does this goal align with the organization?"

Proximal Goals and Roles

Once the overall goal of the team is determined and accepted, the next task is to segment the overarching, distal goal into specific, proximal goals. This includes a breakdown of which roles need to be filled to meet the overall team goals. The research basis for this challenge has been well documented. For example, a study of 31 nursing teams found that the teams with short-term goals (proximal goals) that acted as intermediary steps to accomplishing the overall goal (distal goals) performed better than teams that just focused on the overall goal.[14]

We take this notion one step further, suggesting that leaders consider each overall goal as a series of individual roles that each team member must fill. These roles act as "short-term" goals that are the necessary pieces that have to be completed together to achieve the overall goal.[15] Each role must be filled with people who have the necessary skills, knowledge and ability (often highlighted as SKAs) to succeed.

Let us reiterate. When designing a team, there needs to be a conscious effort to adequately determine the skills, knowledge and abilities needed to succeed in a role, and then match the role with the person who possesses those qualities. Leaders can misstep by overlooking these determinations. As Michael Stevens and Michael Campion explained, there is an "expectation that employees be capable of the technical demands of the job." [16] As a leader, you want to make every effort to secure teammates who have the SKAs needed for success.

Case in point, a practice was attempting to hire a senior surgeon as a reaction to the increased number of surgeries performed by the practice. They identified the critical skills, knowledge and abilities needed to succeed in the surgeon's role. The partners of the practice interviewed several candidates and decided to make the job offer to one candidate with an impeccable surgery record. Yet there was one "ding."

With high patient satisfaction reports, his former colleagues pointed out his immense talent. They also zeroed in on "how much of a pain" it was to work under or with him. His former colleagues noted with understated kindness that "he was not a people person."

Some partners argued that this wasn't really an issue because most of the surgeons acted with a relatively high degree of autonomy. From their consideration of roles, it was more important that the new member be able to perform well and provide patient satisfaction than to interact smoothly with his peers. The firm decided to make him an offer as one of the senior surgeons in the firm.

Then a senior surgeon who had been performing as the team's leader announced her retirement. She was well liked among her colleagues because of her empathetic perspective and her ability to work with the surgeons. The immediate response? The suggestion was made that the new senior surgeon could assume the leadership role. Of course, there was absolutely no evidence that the new surgeon had the needed skills, knowledge and ability for the leadership role, In fact, the contrary seemed more likely.

Including "People" People

Another concept that is important to keep in mind while designing a team is to include "collectivistic" team members. Individuals range in their orientation from individualistic to collectivistic. Our understanding of this concept stems from the studies on country cultures. Some cultures are much more individualistic, while others are more collectivistic. Similarly, within any given culture, individuals within that culture vary in their individualistic versus collectivistic orientation.

Individualistic team members tend to focus on achieving success by themselves. They derive a sense of self-pride from being responsible for success. Conversely, individuals who are collectivistic are much more team oriented. They derive a sense of self-pride from being part of a team that is successful. Not surprisingly, those with collectivistic leanings are much more motivated to work in teams than are those with more individualistic orientations.[17] Further, teams that are composed of collectivistic individuals are less likely to suffer from social loafing.

To maximize individual-level performance, each team member must understand two key points: the overarching goal of the team; and how their individual role plays an important part in reaching the team's overarching goal. As a leader, you can help this occur while engaging team members in a discussion about what they think their individual goals should be. Remember, your goal as the leader is to create buy-in from the followers to the goal while maximizing their skills, knowledge and abilities so that the team accomplishes a task that could not be accomplished by one person. To create the buy-in and to maximize members' efforts, it is important that they believe they have a say in how they can best help accomplish the goal.

There is an additional subtlety. The leader should strive to enhance each team member's "task identity" and "task significance" — both of which help provide greater meaning and purpose of work and lead to higher performance.[18] Task significance refers to the ability to understand the important impact one's task has on others in the organization.[19] Task identity refers to "the ability to complete a whole piece of work."[20] This enhances the meaning of the work being done and can lead to higher performance.[21]

The Role System

Team members should have an accurate virtual role system — a mental schema of all of the roles that must be played in the team and who is filling those roles. Teams are more resilient when they not only understand the virtual role system, but also the need for filling vacated roles.[22] For instance, during performance-focused activity, there is frequently no time to discuss why a team member has vacated a typical role. Instead, adept team members focus on making sure that all the roles are filled so the team can perform.

As a leader, you can facilitate the use of virtual role systems. First, ensure that all the team members understand the various roles that have to be played and who gravitates toward these roles. By having this communication with your followers, they develop clarity in what roles they are expected to play and in who they should anticipate will be filling other roles.

Second, as a leader, you should communicate that you expect that all roles will be filled — asserting that the team should be flexible enough to compensate for momentary changes in role demands. Last, you can demonstrate how a virtual role system is used during performance. That is, when one of your team members is not filling a role during performance, you can step up and play the role so that the team moves forward. The heat of the battle is not the time to reprimand. It is a time of guided action toward accomplishing a goal. There will be time to adjust, fix and guide the team members to improve interactions and exchanges while the team is building its "mental model."

Member Participation in Goal Setting

At the beginning of the previous section, we noted that as a leader you must start with an overarching, distal goal, break that goal down into proximal goals, and then determine the roles that must be filled to accomplish the proximal goals. From there, you design your team based on the skills, knowledge and abilities needed for each role.

Once the team is formed, we suggest that you allow your followers to participate in the goal setting process. Remember that you already have a pretty clear idea of the various goals, but by allowing your team members to participate in goal setting, you are engaging in a form of consultation.

In your mind, you may have already decided the team goals and the various roles that must realistically be engaged. In all honesty, at this point, it can be much easier to set the direction of the team without consulting your team members. In this manner, you avoid the conversation with your followers that may cause leaders anxiety and annoyance as team members disagree with your goal and bring in tangential issues.

We encourage you, though, to engage in the conversation with your team members about setting team goals, and in turn setting the individuals goals of each team member. There is an empirically sound reason for this. When individuals are involved with goal setting, they are much more likely to accept the goal and put in more effort to accomplishing that goal.[23] However, you do not want to allow team members free rein in setting goals because they may set goals that are not consistent with your vision and the needed direction.[24] You want your followers to be involved in goal setting, but you want to make sure that you guide the process and align their individual needs and goals to the vision that you have.

Mental Models

Mental models can be conceptualized as an individual's understanding of the strategies that work.[25] We develop mental models all the time. For instance, you were probably trained how to determine if a patient was a drug seeker. If a patient complains of nonspecific pain and asks for a narcotic by name, your antennae go up and a mental model is activated.

Team mental models are the collective understanding of what a team must do to perform at a high level. Teams that have an accurate, shared team mental model have higher performance.[26] These are termed "shared mental models" when they are understood by team members.[27] John Mathieu and others explain that when team mental models are shared, team members "will easily coordinate their actions and be in sync."[28]

The points noted above present an additional reason why long-standing, intact teams tend to outperform newly formed teams. Stated simply, they have had time to build, accept and share accurate team mental models. As a leader, though, you can manage the process of building an accurate, shared team mental model, thus helping your team reach higher performance more quickly than what would occur through natural time together.

To build an accurate and shared team mental model, the leader should guide the team through several steps.[29] Initially, you can prime the team that one of the goals is to focus and try to determine the accurate team mental model. That is, before your team performs a task, you ask your team members to try to consciously figure out the "strategy for winning teamwork" while they are doing the task. After the group performs a task, hold a debriefing session — a postmortem, if you will — that includes two steps. Engage the team members in a discussion, with each member recognizing something the team did that was good — i.e., elements of the team mental model that were accurate. Next, engage the team in a discussion to identify the errors — where the team might not have had perfect performance, areas for improvement or where breakdowns occurred. Finally, based on what is revealed, engage members in a discussion about what they believe to be the accurate team mental model, and, as a group, devise a strategy for their next performance.

High-performing teams do not stop here, though. They repeat this process over and over. This process becomes so routine and ingrained into the team that the discussions begin to just happen. In high-performing teams, these types of discussions are ongoing and productive. As a leader, you can encourage a culture that engages in team mental model building by informally asking your team members about what they think needs to be done to improve the team.

There is one additional nuance with team mental model building for many physicians. The research shows that long-standing teams usually outperform temporary teams because they build accurate, shared team mental models that allow them to anticipate the actions of fellow team members so the co-ordination of the team is very fluid.[30]

Team Efficacy

You will recall that efficacy is the belief that you can accomplish something. In like manner, team efficacy arises when individual members believe in the team's ability to reach an assigned goal.[31] With high team efficacy, members tend to set higher goals and are more likely to try again in the face of setbacks than are teams with low team efficacy.[32]

Building team efficacy is similar to how one builds self-efficacy — through verbal persuasion, vicarious experiences and mastery. We encourage leaders of a new team to work on all three in order. Start by verbally affirming your own individual belief in the team's capability. Then, if you are able, provide examples of peer teams that have succeeded. Finally, look for "low hanging fruit," goals that you think would be easily accomplishable. Make the goal known and when it is reached acknowledge it.

When Teams Break Down

One of the more interesting and popular looks at teams has come from Patrick Lencioni in his best-selling book *The Five Dysfunctions of a Team*.[33] Lencioni contends that when teams fail to meet their potential, one or more of five team themes or pitfalls is probably occurring. These pitfalls or team dysfunctions are depicted in Table 5.1. They are an absence of trust, a fear of conflict, a lack of commitment, avoidance of accountability and inattention to results. Logically, team functionality must embrace the positive dimensions of these five themes.

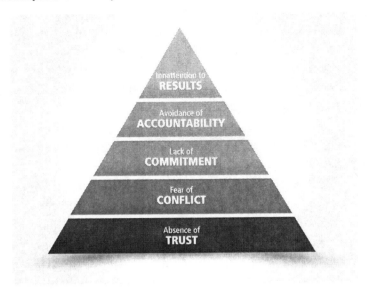

Table 5.1

Importantly, Lencioni states that these five themes occur in a hier-archical or successive manner — that is, trust precedes a willingness to openly engage in conflict, which precedes a depth of commitment, which is foundational for meaningful accountability, which fosters performance results. He notes that a team breakdown at one level will eventuate into problems at the next level. Stated slightly differently, when we experience a breakdown in one level, it is most likely because of a problem with some preceding level or step.

Let's clarify the somewhat obvious but quite practical impact. We often encounter intact teams that, by their own admission, are struggling with commitment, accountability and results. Digging deep, we typically find that unresolved issues of trust and conflict are the likely culprits. The presence of team trust and respectful conflict will not guarantee subsequent commitment, accountability and results. However, deficiencies in trust and conflict will generally manifest as breakdowns of commitment, accountability and action.

It is probably not surprising that Lencioni has zeroed in on "distrust" as the basis for most dysfunctional teams. Predictably, we know that teams that experience high levels of member trust perform better than teams that are filled with distrust.[34]

There are certain fundamental behaviors that should be stressed. Of course, respect must be a front-burner issue, and a tone of interactional respect must be assured. But there must be more. Trust means that members can be open and vulnerable, admitting when they do not understand and when they need help. These admissions must be met with a developmental spirit and never derision. Team members must support one another within and without the team context. Members must feel that others "have their back." In turn, members are more willing to share openly and take risks.[35]

Let us examine a situation that one physician faced. This physician, board certified in emergency medicine, worked a 24-hour shift. At 4 a.m., 20 hours into the shift, she sees a young mother with a 2-year-old with a fever. The young mother explained that she was at her primary care physician earlier in the day but he just told her that the child had a viral infection and to use Tylenol to reduce the fever. She followed the orders and gave the child his last dose at 9 p.m. before he fell asleep. When the child woke at 3 a.m. crying, the fever had returned. The young mother explained to the ER doctor that "I just know there is something more wrong. I think my baby needs antibiotics."

The physician listened to the mother with empathy, examined the child and patiently explained, "There is good news. Your child is going to be fine. He has a viral infection, just as your physician diagnosed, and I also recommend to continue with the prescribed treatment. You are doing everything right and your child is going to be fine."

Although sensing that the mother was not completely satisfied, she left the mother to complete the patient satisfaction survey. Although the mother did not write any negative comments, she did check "No" to the question "Were you satisfied with your experience in the ER?" The physician finished her 24-hour shift at 8 a.m. and went to sleep for a few hours before closing out her charts. When she returned to the ER to finish her paperwork for her shift, the director of the ER was at the nurses' station.

As the exhausted physician approached, the ER director said, "What the hell happened here last night? We had a complaint that a patient wasn't satisfied?" The physician, a little taken aback, started to present the case to the director. Before she was able to get far, the director raised his voice so that all in earshot could hear, "This is unacceptable. We expect 100 percent patient satisfaction!" before storming off. The physician was left standing with all eyes on her in disbelief at the lack of respect her director had shown to her — in front of the staff that she had to lead.

There are many issues that we could discuss with this story. We could dive into the director's unrealistic expectations for his physicians (i.e., 100 percent satisfaction rate), or how this was a vivid, object lesson in how not to deal with conflict. But here we would like to focus on the impact of the director's actions on trust.

The physician explained, "I just felt so humiliated. I had done everything right. I know I had. I practiced good medicine, and perhaps more important, I tried to be empathetic and compassionate to the patient. I accept that I can't satisfy all patients. But the humiliating part was the questioning of my decisions as a leader — the questioning of my ability in front of the team of staff that I have to lead. I felt that they were now going to doubt me. I felt in that one act, the director undermined the authority I need and put a dent in the 10 years I've worked to have a relationship with my staff."

Maybe she was overly sensitive from lack of sleep. Maybe she's just overly sensitive in general, making this incident seem bigger than it was. But, in a sense, she is right, and her concern seems well placed. Even if some discussion was needed, the method of derisiveness and the public nature of the exchange will likely make other members of the staff be tentative — wondering when their turn may come. The lack of trust, coupled with disrespect, even turned a productive team toxic, rippling with waves of distrust that may slow the delivery of care and limit critical patient outcomes.

How does she repair the trust that may have been broken with her staff? First, let's look at the basic psychology of trust.

Conceptually, there are two related yet different types of trust.[36] First, "cognitive trust" refers to trust by observation. That is, we observe others and draw a conclusion based on our perceptions of whether there is consistency in the behaviors and actions. If colleagues say they are going to do something, and then they do it, we start to trust that person's word. This is cognitive trust.

Cognitive trust is surface trust, essentially trust that individuals must verify. However, once cognitive trust has been established, we progress to a second and deeper level, known as "affective trust."

Affective trust is based on an emotional connection, almost a liking. Once affective trust is built, it creates a much stronger bond than cognitive trust. When individuals are in the cognitive trust stage of a relationship, a single act of mistrust can seriously harm the trust between two people. However, once affective trust is built, then any one act of mistrust usually does not breach the long-term trust between the two parties (of course, this depends on the severity of the violation of the mistrust).

Fortunately, since the ER physician had built trust (affective trust) over a period of years, her team was able to experience the recent explosion from a more refined and balanced perspective. The physician continued to work hard. She maintained the high level of standards she always had. Consequently, the nurses forgot about the incident, instead focusing on the number of times the physician did follow through with conviction.

Bricolage

Well-known professor of management Karl Weick described how to make small teams more resilient when they are operating in quickly changing environments.[37] His work has increased relevance as we face situations that are so unfamiliar that we have no immediate ability to make sense of them.

Weick has encouraged teams to engage in the process of bricolage — a term that literally implies activities of "tinkering." Bricolage occurs when team members are able to "make do" with elements they have at hand, adapting and adjusting so that they can implement strategies that work despite having limited resources. Bricolage creates a powerful mindset for teams. Bricolage encourages adaptation, flexibility and consideration of seemingly unrelated knowledge and ideas, all with an eye toward moving forward in the face of uncertainty and even panic.

Leaders set the tone that allows bricolage to arise and flourish. A willingness to adapt initial strategies is key. Encourage your teams to use the resources at hand. Encourage flexibility. Instead of "entertaining the panic," a good leader helps the team focus on what is the same, what changes need to be made because of situational differences, and how current resources can be adapted and used to overcome the situational differences.

Communication

Communication is the key to high-performing teams. Team members talk to each other, and they talk often. Team members must talk openly and honestly to build a mutual understanding of each other's needs while performing teamwork. Communication is fundamental to building an accurate shared team mental model.

First, let's consider the different types of messages that have to be communicated. There are some communications that are purely conveyance, which is sharing information with others. Other communications are convergence. These are conversations where both parties must share ideas to come to a new mutual understanding.

At the same time, communication channels — our methods of communication — range in their richness. The richest communication channel is face-to-face communication. At the other end, a lean communication channel would be email. Research has shown that for conveyance messages, leaner communication channels are perfectly fine, and in fact, perhaps better.[38] Conversely, if convergence messages are trying to be communicated, richer communication channels are necessary.

We have all been in the situation where we are engaged in email discussions. Individuals write longer and longer responses with more tangents in their retorts. In this case, a richer communication channel is needed. Rule of thumb, email your team members if you want to share information; meet with them if you need to build a new mutual understanding.

The communication patterns and interactions of high-performing teams also vary from those of low-performing teams.[39] High-performing teams communicate much more frequently than low-performing teams. Further, when they do meet, they speak in short, concise statements, making logical points, and the team members speak in roughly equal amounts. They speak with excitement and engagement when they communicate with their teammates.

The point of an equal amount of sharing is important. As the leader, it is important that you take charge of the meeting, in that you have an idea of the issues that are necessary to discuss and to keep the conversation on point. However, as a leader, it is also your responsibility to allow the team members to talk. Research on leader dialogue has shown that leaders who talk disproportionally more than their followers in the team give the perception that the leader is not open to discussion or alternative ideas. As a result, the followers in the team tend to share less information, resulting in lower team performance.[40]

Meeting Mania

Within contemporary organizations, few topics elicit more frustration than meetings. It may seem that much of your administrative role is simply rotating from one meeting to another. Often, meetings provoke a strange sense of déjà vu. "This seems like the same meeting we had last week." And, of course, we fear that we will probably have this meeting again next week. Time, talent and resources are consumed, and progress comes at a glacial pace.

This visceral negativity toward meetings need not be present. Generally, poor meetings result from one of three factors: poor planning, ineffective leadership or nonexistent follow-up.

The first question regarding meetings deals with the need for and propriety of holding the meeting. In short, does this meeting really need to take place? Or, is there a legitimate reason for this meeting? The fact that it is on the schedule is insufficient. Your team members are under time constraints. If the only purpose of the meeting is to transfer information, perhaps a leaner channel can be used.

However, we must never diminish the times when meetings are needed. When we need to explore, discuss, share interpretations and make decisions, we should meet. When we need to build relationships and rapport, we should meet. When there is an unacceptable risk of misinterpretation, we should meet. When we need assurance that everyone is on the same page and supportive of our actions, we should meet. When emotional undertones are present, we should meet.

Once we determine that a meeting has legitimacy, our concern turns to efficiency. Many of the topics and themes of this chapter come crisply into play. However, there are other specific actions that may be helpful.

First, consider the amount of time that should be allotted to meetings and carefully time-limit your meetings. In a clinical setting, a regular staff meeting could be quite brief. Cross-functional, administrative meetings will surely run longer. Yet, even here, we encourage team leaders to think in one-hour blocks of time. Beyond this, attention wanes and distractions intensify. Of course, we understand that issues may, at times, demand larger blocks of time. However, these should be viewed as exceptions rather than the rule.

Distributing an agenda at least one day before the meeting helps members prepare and organize their thoughts. Accordingly, agendas facilitate team efficiency. The agenda should signify priority of discussion and may even include time suggestions per agenda item. As we all know, the items on the agenda tend to expand to fit the time allotted. Early items almost always yield more intense discussion and higher levels of involvement. Plan accordingly.

The leader must allow team members a range of flexibility while adhering to the agenda items. Some team members will be perennial "wanderers," taking the team off on side roads or launching into irrelevant "war stories." The leader must respectfully bring the team back to the agenda.

A summary should be prepared and distributed to team members within 24 hours of the meeting's close. This summary should highlight the decisions that were made, the actions that will take place and the items to be considered before the next meeting. In this way, the summary carries motivational impact — showing people clearly what the meeting accomplished. Further, the summary sets the tone for subsequent meetings, thereby building momentum and continuity.

Concluding Thoughts: Disengaged Team Members

A disengaged team member is one who does not buy into the teamwork mentality. We experience levels of disengagement ranging from active to passive. Passively disengaged team members exhibit certain patterns. They show up; they participate; and they do their teamwork. However, their effort is minimal to the point of just getting by.

Conversely, actively disengaged team members are social loafers. They withdraw and they create conflict in the team. These team members miss key performance deadlines. Often, they are verbally combative to team initiatives. They create demonstrative acts of team subterfuge by interacting with their phones during meetings rather than their colleagues.

Addressing these individuals is always challenging. We may need to help them see the value and impact of the team's efforts. We may have to help them reprioritize. Or we may need to have a tough, honest and respectful conflict encounter — the topic of our next chapter.

1. http://www.phoenix.edu/news/releases/2013/01/university-of-phoenix-survey-reveals-nearly-seven-in-ten-workers-have-been-part-of-dysfunctional-teams.html

2. Sundstrom, E., De Meuse, K.P., & Futrell, D. (1990). Work teams: Applications and effectiveness. *American Psychologist, 45(2),* 120-133.

3. Katzenbach, J.R., & Smith, D.K. (1993). *The Wisdom of Teams: Creating the high-performance organization.* McKinsey and Co. *Inc.,* USA, 113-116.

4. Zaponc, R. (1965). Social facilitation. *Science, 149,* 269-274.

5. Karau, S.J. & Williams, K.D. (1993). Social loafing: A meta-analytic review and theoretical integration. *Journal of Personality and Social Psychology, 65(4),* 681-706.

6. Tuckman, B.W., & Jensen, M.A.C. (1977). Stages of small-group development revisited. *Group & Organization Management, 2(4),* 419-427.

7. Hackman, R. (1987). The design of work teams. In J. Lorsch (ed.), *Handbook of Organizational Behavior* (pp. 315-342). Upper Saddle River, NJ: Prentice Hall.

8. http://humanresources.about.com/od/teambuildingfaqs/f/optimum-team-size.htm

9. Carron, A. V., Spink, K. S., & Prapavessis, H. (1997). Team building and cohesiveness in the sport and exercise setting: Use of indirect interventions. *Journal of Applied Sport Psychology, 9(1),* 61-72.

10. Katzenbach, J.R. & Smith, D.K. (1993). *The Wisdom of Teams: Creating the high-performance organization.* New York: Harper, p. xix.

11. Hackman, R. & Staats, B. (2013). The hidden benefits of keeping teams intact. *Harvard Business Review, 91*(12), 27-29.

12. Ibid., p. 196.

13. Ibid., p. 27-29.

14. Weldon, E., & Yun, S. (2000). The effects of proximal and distal goals on goal level, strategy development and group performance. *The Journal of Applied Behavioral Science, 36(3),* 336-344.

15. Stone, P., & Veloso, M. (1999). Task decomposition, dynamic role assignment, and low-bandwidth communication for real-time strategic teamwork. *Artificial Intelligence, 110(2),* 241-273.

16. Stevens, M.J., & Campion, M.A. (1994). The knowledge, skill, and ability requirements for teamwork: Implications for human resource management. *Journal of Management, 20(2),* 503-530.

17. Shaw, J.D., Duffy, M.K., & Stark, E. M. (2000). Interdependence and preference for group work: Main and congruence effects on the satisfaction and performance of group members. *Journal of Management, 26(2),* 259-279.

18. Cummings, T.G. (1978). Self-regulating work groups: A socio-technical synthesis. *Academy of Management Review, 3(3),* 625-634.

19. Hackman, J.R., & Oldham, G.R. (1975). Development of the job diagnostic survey. *Journal of Applied Psychology, 60(2),* 159 –170. Morgeson, F.P., & Humphrey, S.E. (2006). The Work Design Questionnaire (WDQ): Developing and validating a comprehensive measure for assessing job design and the nature of work. *Journal of Applied Psychology, 91(6),* 1321–1339.

20. Cummings T.G. (1978). Self-regulating work groups: A socio-technical synthesis. *Academy of Management Review, 3(3),* 625-634.

21. Berg, J. M., Dutton, J. E., & Wrzesniewski, A. (2013). Job crafting and meaningful work. In B.J. Dik, Z.S. Byrne & M.F. Steger (Eds.), *Purpose and Meaning in the Workplace* (pp. 81-104). Washington, D.C.: American Psychological Association. Grant, A.M. (2007). Relational job design and the motivation to make a prosocial difference. *Academy of Management Review, 32(2)*, 393-417. Grant, A.M. (2008). The significance of task significance: Job performance effects, relational mechanisms, and boundary conditions. *Journal of Applied Psychology, 93(1)*, 108-124. Grant, A.M., & Parker, S.K. (2009). Redesigning work design theories: The rise of relational and proactive perspectives. *Academy of Management Annals, 3(1)*, 317-375.

22. Weick, Karl E. (1993). The collapse of sensemaking in organizations: The Mann Gulch disaster. *Administrative Science Quarterly, 38,(4),* 628-652.

23. Erez, M.P., Earley, C., & Hulin, C.L. (1985). The impact of participation on goal acceptance and performance: A two-step model. *Academy of Management Journal, 28(1)*, 50-66.

24. Schneider, B., Brief, A.P., & Guzzo, R.A. (1996). Creating a climate and culture for sustainable organizational change. *Organizational Dynamics, 24*(4), 7-19.

25. Mohammed, S., & Dumville, B.C. (2001). Team mental models in a team knowledge framework: Expanding theory and measurement across disciplinary boundaries. *Journal of Organizational Behavior, 22(2)*, 89-106.

26. Lim, B. & Klein, K.J. (2006). Team mental models and team performance: a field study of the effects of team mental model similarity and accuracy. *Journal of Organizational Behavior, 27(4)*, 403-418.

27. Mathieu, J.E., Heffner, T.S., Goodwin, G.F., Salas, E., & Cannon-Bowers, J.A. (2000). The influence of shared mental models on team process and performance. *Journal of Applied Psychology, 85(2)*, 273-283.

28. Mathieu, J.E., Heffner, T.S., Goodwin, G.F., Salas, E., & Cannon-Bowers, J.A. (2000). The influence of shared mental models on team process and performance. *Journal of Applied Psychology, 85(2)*, 273-283.

29. Smith-Jentsch, K.A., Cannon-Bowers, J.A., Tannenbaum, S. I., & Salas, E. (2008). Guided team self-correction impacts on team mental models, processes, and effectiveness. *Small Group Research, 39(3)*, 303-327.

30. Katz, R. (1982). The effects of group longevity on project communication and performance. *Administrative Science Quarterly, 27(1)*, 81-104. Pfeffer, J. (1983). Organizational demography. *Research in Organizational Behavior, 5,* 299-357.

31. Gully, S.M., Incalcaterra, K.A., Joshi, A., & Beaubien, J.M. (2002). A meta-analysis of team-efficacy, potency, and performance: interdependence and level of analysis as moderators of observed relationships. *Journal of Applied Psychology, 87(5)*, 819-832.

32. Gibson, C.B. (1999). Do they do what they believe they can? Group efficacy and group effectiveness across tasks and cultures. *Academy of Management Journal, 42(2)*, 138–152.

33. Lencioni, P. (2002). *The Five Dysfunctions of a Team.* San Francisco: Jossey-Bass.

34. Erdem, F., & Ozen, J. (2003). Cognitive and affective dimensions of trust in developing team performance. *Team Performance Management: An International Journal, 9(5/6)*, 131-135.

35. Lencioni, P. (2002). *The Five Dysfunctions of a Team.* San Francisco: Jossey-Bass.

36. Mayer, R.C., Davis, J. H., & Schoorman, F.D. (1995). An integrative model of organizational trust. *Academy of Management Review, 20(3)*, 709-734.

37. Weick, K.E. (1993). The collapse of sensemaking in organizations: The Mann Gulch disaster. *Administrative Science Quarterly, 38(4),* 628-652.

38. Dennis, A.R., & Valacich, J.S. (1999). Rethinking media richness: Toward a theory of media synchronicity. In *Systems Sciences, 1999. HICSS-32. Proceedings of the 32nd Annual Hawaii International Conference on.* IEEE.

39. Pentland, A. S. (2012). The new science of building great teams. *Harvard Business Review,* April, 60-70.

40. Tost, L.P., Gino, F., & Larrick, R.P. (2013) When power makes others speechless: The negative impact of leader power on team performance. *Academy of Management Journal, 56(5),* 1465-1486.

6

Conflict: The Power of
Respectful Conflict Encounters

···

PHYSICIANS WORK IN COMPLICATED SETTINGS LADEN WITH A MAZE of interlocking needs. Even in situations where all parties readily agree on the eventual goal of patient well-being, it is likely that professional experts, each seeking to fulfill the unique norms and viewpoints of their disciplines, will differ on the proper course of action.[1] And, of course, perspectives grow with the complexity of the patient's condition. We know, in both intuitive and practical ways, that these divergent views must be "reconciled and integrated — a need that has become more acute as both the degree of subspecialization and the diversity of care team members increases."[2]

You are now experiencing additional challenges that arise from working closely with both clinical and nonclinical leaders whose goals, agendas and approaches vary and clash. To further exacerbate the situation, each party has a compelling opinion that is bolstered by a foundation of specialized expertise. And, as if these smoldering embers needed any additional spark, each party communicates in a language coded with idiosyncrasies.

Senior leadership pursues its own set of performance metrics. Finance and accounting leaders speak of cost containment, return on investment and operating margins — all the while seemingly minimizing our central patient focus. Add in our Six Sigma project representatives, whose carefully prescribed regimen of feasibility assessments will certainly add an extra year of study to an obvious need that should be addressed today.

From these and countless other sources, conflict seems inevitable. And it is. We laud the need for congruence, unity and generally accepted best practices. And what we get is conflict — a condition that is certain and natural. As we will discuss in this chapter, the concern is not the presence of conflict, but what we do with it — how we experience it, how we handle it, how we grow from it — to enable and enhance our work rather than diminish it.

The Upside of Conflict

We begin with an assertion that every successful leader understands and accepts, at least from an intellectual perspective. While conflict may present discomfort and interpersonal tensions, it is an absolutely essential factor for success in today's fast-paced, change-focused world. There are at least four reasons for this assertion.

First, we have long accepted that conflict is the spark for meaningful innovation. For example, in his classic work *Innovation and Entrepreneurship*, Peter Drucker recognized that one of the prompts or opportunities for innovation comes from incongruity — a conflict between some desired and needed state of outcomes and current reality.[3] In essence, conflict becomes the inflection point for creative reconsideration of processes and approaches that generate meaningful innovation.[4]

There is a second, closely related issue. Without conflict, change would be unlikely. For example, experts have argued that leaders should be "creating a motivation to change" by demonstrating a sense of disruption or disconfirmation — intentionally injecting forces of tension and conflict to rattle people from the status quo.[5] Edgar Schein has even stretched leaders to recognize that such disconfirmation can thrust organizational members into a state of "survival anxiety," an urgent awareness that change must occur or "something bad will happen."[6]

Within the context of both innovation and change, conflict discussions are expansive. That is, open consideration of one area of conflict often leads to deeper discussions revealing additional awareness and need. Here, leaders can employ "opportunity thinking," recognizing that conflict, when recognized and addressed, often yields opportunities for necessary growth and competitive realignment.

Third, conflict provides an essential system of checks and balances. We are bombarded by daily reminders of unchecked malfeasance because of underprescribed oversight. These examples range from corporate heights to individual movements and cover nearly any context we can imagine. But the idea of checks and balances is more deeply strategic than it is moral and legal. Visionary leaders are often reservoirs of novel ideas and creative initiatives. Many of these ideas push others in important and needed directions. Yet these meritorious ideas often need to be massaged and tweaked for maximum impact. In some cases, seemingly amazing ideas may even need to be delayed or abandoned. Encouraging dissenting perspectives and conflicting views is one of the best ways to ensure that we do not veer off into dangerous or unwarranted territory.

We work with a CEO who is one of the most creative and innovative people we have ever met. Stylistically, he is an off-the-charts innovator, producing a steady stream of opportunistic initiatives and projects. His executive staff, by design, is considerably more conservative. In fact, the CEO expects and demands that his most trusted staff members "shoot holes in his ideas." He has learned that without staff pushback the risk of taking a "half-baked idea to market" is just too high. In a way, the conflict that others interject provides the CEO the freedom to be more expansive and push more boundaries in his thinking.

Fourth, when conflict is addressed directly and respectfully, it has the potential to enhance interpersonal connections, deepen trust, and foster a dynamic and progressive organizational culture.[7] We are reminded of Fred Jandt's poignant words, "A relationship in conflict *is* a relationship — not the absence of one.[8]

When conflict is addressed openly, it can prompt creative inquiry that leads to status-quo- breaking innovations and progressive organizational growth.[9] Conflict forces us to challenge established patterns and approaches, many of which have become stale, outdated and irrelevant.

The Downside

Nevertheless, most of us do not energetically cherish the opportunity to embrace conflict and engage in a theoretically advantageous but pragmatically uncomfortable situation. Many people recoil at the prospect of impending conflict, going out of their way to avoid the potentially ugly entanglements that accompany pointed interpersonal exchanges. Not surprisingly, evidence suggests that the prevailing leadership approach when faced with troubling interpersonal conflict is avoidance.[10]

At the other end of the conflict continuum we see leaders who rush in boldly, confronting the issues and people, employing a take-no-prisoners style in the process. Dissenters are beaten, intellectually and emotionally, into submission.

In some cases, avoidance may be an appropriate option, especially when it is the product of strategic positioning rather than mere capitulation. Some situations do work out with time. Further, some situations should be avoided temporarily or postponed: when factual clarity is needed (information or evidence needs to be gathered or expanded) or the emotional arousal of the parties suggests that an immediate confrontation would be imprudent and counterproductive.

However, most cases of avoidance are not the product of such thoughtful cognitive deliberations. Instead, leaders sense that the conversation should take place but opt for the safety of delay. Given all the critical episodes and decisions you encounter each day, it is easy to understand why one would not choose to divert time and emotional energy toward the uncertainty of a conflict encounter. Recognize that such delays carry three significant costs. First, a troubling situation is perpetuated. Second, as others become aware of your unwillingness to address the issue, feelings of inequity and injustice may arise. And third, inactivity may be a threat to the leader's credibility.

Litigious concerns aside, most leaders avoid needed conflict encounters because of perceived skill deficiency, leading to a low sense of confidence in one's capacity to engage in a tough conversation (that is laden with emotion) without causing deeper damage.[11] One of the goals of this chapter is to help you build skill and confidence in engaging in respectful conflict encounters.

Resolving or Managing Conflict

When we think of conflict, we conjure images of differences in attitude and stance due to divergent points of view and contradictory needs. Given the likely volume of such divergence, pragmatism demands that we consider whether we should attempt to resolve an immediate, presenting conflict; or alternatively seek to manage it. Each approach has a different goal.

Conflict management strives for "a state of uniformity or convergence of purpose or means; conflict management only realigns the divergence enough to render the opposing forces less diametrically opposite and damaging to each other."[12] Conflict management erects buffers so that the destructive components of conflict can be mitigated.

On the other hand, conflict resolution requires that we dig into the issues, understand the underlying needs, and structure solutions that ease immediate tensions and diminish the likelihood of recurrence. While this chapter focuses on conflict resolution as an underdeveloped leadership competency, we understand that conflict management is the prudent choice in some situations.

There are at least two situational factors that angle in favor of management over resolution. The first is time. The second is prioritization. Generally, resolution requires more time than management. In contexts where immediate decisions are needed and delay is costly, conflict management may be the more prudent option. Prioritization follows a similar path. Here, we have so many critical issues to address that exhausting energy on resolution is not the best deployment of our time or resources.

Buffering or separating the conflicting parties to minimize interactional opportunities can be a low-cost, short-term approach.

At times, we can use creative "bridge strategies" to create a linkage and crossover between conflict management and conflict resolution. One of the more interesting and well-studied approaches is the use of the superordinate goal that can applied to teams as well as individuals. The original idea of the superordinate goals came from the work of Muzafer and Carolyn Sherif's Robbers Cave experiments.[13] Researchers found that if conflicting groups were forced to interact, conflict did not abate. However, by injecting a superordinate goal things changed.

A superordinate goal must meet two conditions. First, it must be a goal that is important to the conflicting factions. Second, the goal must be attainable only if the factions agree to work together. Note that the intent here is not to resolve the underlying issues but only to create a condition where factions must work together, for specific periods of time, to achieve mutually desired outcomes.

Let's be clear, when faced with a superordinate goal, factions cooperated only because they felt they had to, in essence perceiving a state of emergency necessitating interaction and cooperation. And it is certainly possible that once the immediate emergency is averted, battle lines are redrawn and conflict proceeds unabated. However, another outcome is also possible. Research found that as conflicting parties interacted, shared sentiments with one another and experienced the exposure of some unwarranted biases, the actual bases of the underlying conflict were dissipated.

The Structure of Interpersonal Conflict

There are many sources of interpersonal conflict. At times, it arises because of the competitive and highly politicized nature of our organizational environments, as well-intentioned people battle over limited resources. At times, conflicts arise when multiple parties examine the same evidence and garner divergent views of both meaning and implication — no doubt heavily influenced by personal and team agendas. At times, personality and stylistic differences foster interpersonal antagonism that amplifies relatively minor points of disconnect. Despite these rather obvious precipitating factors, there is a more basic level. Consider the following example.

In her early 40s, Lei Hardy had built a solid reputation based on both outstanding clinical skills and an aggressive research agenda. Hardy brought several junior faculty members into her research projects. One of those projects, studying the use of "intact surgical teams and outcome quality" even received national attention. As principal investigator on this research, Hardy included two junior faculty members and secured a $50,000 grant.

Late last spring, buoyed by the prospects and potential of her research, Hardy approached her dean, requesting 20 percent release time to devote to her research. The request seemed reasonable given that others had received research release time and that colleagues encouraged her to proceed with the request. Given Hardy's past work and productivity, the dean agreed that the request had merit and said he would try to honor her request. Two months later, the dean affirmed the value of Hardy's work but noted that further consideration for her request would have to be delayed until the next budget period. Hardy, while disappointed, agreed to the delay largely because of the wave of changes that were taking place within the hospital.

A bit later, the dean informed Hardy that the release time could not be honored during the current fiscal year. The dean cited cost concerns and heightened attention to faculty clinical activities as his rationale. Hardy was both surprised and clearly disappointed. From her perspective, the denial meant an inevitable lag in the research, reducing the timeliness of the work. It also would require a rather significant overhaul of her planned workload.

Hardy asked her dean for a meeting to address this conflict, and it was a meeting laden with landmines. The relationship between the dean and Hardy had always been cordial and professional but certainly not warm. In fact, Hardy heard through the rumor mill that the dean had expressed to others that Hardy was "a prima donna more interested in personal aggrandizement than being a team player." It is not hard to imagine the emotional intensity that was dripping from this encounter.

Here, we encounter conflict's pivotal issue. Most of us begin to sense or experience interpersonal conflict when our expectations — which are reasonable and realistic because they are ours — are dashed or blocked by another party's behavior or lack of behavior. In Hardy's case, her expectation of release time was thwarted, and in her mind, the culprit was the dean. Now one can argue that Hardy's expectations were unfounded, that the dean provided no promise or confirmation. We realize, of course, that this was not Hardy's perspective. In the language of interpersonal conflict, the dean's decision and Hardy's awareness of dashed expectation is specified as the "trigger event." The trigger event activates what follows.

Let's digress to consider another important theoretical point. In his pioneering work, Morton Deutsch distinguished the "manifest conflict" from the "underlying conflict."[14] While terminology has shifted over the years, we prefer the clarity of Deutsch's original designations. The manifest conflict is what we see on the surface, the immediate issue that is present. The underlying conflict is deeper and often hidden. It involves perceptions of power plays, individual value and issues of trust.

The mental processing and behavioral patterns that follow the immediate trigger are predictable. Frustrated by dashed expectations, Hardy begins an adventure of cognitive sifting. Armed with her facts, which are always incomplete, she begins to grasp for interpretations or attributions of causality for what has just occurred.

It will not be a surprise that two facts and an "assumed" fact dominated her attributions: Others have received release time, I have been denied release time and the dean has labeled me a prima donna. Hardy's interpretation will come as no surprise. She asserted that "the dean has it in for me, diminishes my contribution and treats me unfairly." Of course, as the interpretive process unfurls, personal emotions are activated and heightened arousal evolves. In Hardy's case, the most fitting expression of her emotion was anger. Keep in mind that this iterative process unfurls in rapid succession, as our facts lead to our interpretations, prompting our unique emotions and levels of arousal and leading to our actions.[15]

Of course, this rapid succession of events involving limited facts, leading to expedient interpretations and emotional arousal, are the precursors for taking action. Hardy's discussion with the dean was heated and intense, with harsh words, animated exchanges and bitter accusations. By her own admission, Hardy said things she wished she had not said. Of course, once these actions have been expressed, there is no "do-over." And the conflict encounter has led to an expansion rather than reduction in the level of conflict intensity.

Again, research has helped us gain a deeper understanding of these processes. For example, psychologists have delineated two related but contradictory mental structures known as the "hot system" and the "cool system."[16] Located in the amygdala, the hot system is emotional, simple, reflexive and fast. Activated by perceived threats, it prompts the familiar "fight or flight syndrome." Located in the prefrontal cortex, the cool system is rational, complex, slow and cognitively centered and "encourages us to stop and think."[17] Critically, it appears that under stress, the hot system is activated and correspondingly, the cool system is suppressed.[18]

Let's pause for a moment. Knowing that she has a temper and a rather "short fuse," Hardy entered the conflict encounter determined to keep her emotions in check and temper her responses in a judicious manner. In short, she demanded self-control and generated as much focused self-talk to that end as she could muster. In this regard, she was unsuccessful. Yet her behavior is not unexpected. Most of us engage in a rather consistent and habitual pattern of conflict-induced behavior, generally without much regard for its success or lack of success in previous encounters.

This happens largely because of the emotionally aroused hot system impact that we experience and our inability to enact the necessary control checks. In short, we are not making fundamentally rational and strategic decisions. We are making emotional decisions. Some of us are better at filtering and regulating our emotions. Others, like Hardy, are not.

So why are some better at this than others? Three factors seem to be at play: our personal styles or preferences for dealing with conflict; our capacity to flex — to apply different behaviors and styles within the situational demands of conflict, and our established and deeply personal habits.

Working with Hardy, we began to unpack the conflict event and the conflict encounter. First, it is always important to keep reminding ourselves that "our facts" are generally not "all the facts." We are always cognizant that the proverbial "other side of the story" generally looks quite different. Second, Hardy's situation exemplifies the importance of identifying, sharing and clarifying expectations. Recognize that this event hinges on Hardy's perception of broken expectations, a view that may not be shared by the dean.

We cannot stop the precipitating factors or trigger events of conflict. These are part of our interactions and are inherent in organizational life. We can, to some extent, alter our perceptions of these events. Likewise, it is extremely hard to temper the immediacy and reality of quick emotional arousal. But the cause is not hopeless. In any event, Hardy's example helps us begin to understand the need to recognize conflict, understand the dynamics involved and begin to consider behavioral responses that may be helpful.

We return to the importance and power of self-regulation, or more fully the failure of self-regulation, which experts have been described as "the major social pathology of our time."[19] Let's look at some behavioral responses.

The Behaviors of Respectful Conflict Encounters

Selective Avoidance

The first behavior is actually a repressed behavior — the decision to let the conflict go without encounter. We must be quick to add that this selective avoidance response is a strategic and carefully discerned decision, not an act of capitulation born of fear or laziness.

As a young professor, I had the opportunity to work with a wonderful senior leader as we led graduate students through an intense, experientially based course in organizational behavior. The professor was always careful and gentle as he offered advice. With apologies to Mark Twain, as I aged, his wisdom became even more apparent and impressive. Early in our work together, the professor listened as I mused about my frustration with a relatively minor decision. He offered only this: "There are times when it's best to let some things go."

I was reminded of this exchange nearly 20 years later when a senior surgeon described a younger colleague's interpersonal struggles with the staff and other physicians. "Everything is a battle. He makes an issue out of everything." With only minimal sarcasm, the unfortunate reality for both me and the young surgeon was that we both truly believed that our views were right — and frankly, most often they were.

Within this realm there are two points to consider: letting it go and postponing — letting it go for now. We choose to let things go because the events do not rise to a threshold that warrants further intensification. The issues are small; the impact is minimal; the risks are low; the outcomes are only slightly and inconsequentially affected and the likelihood of problematic escalation is low.

There is also another situation where we should let go — to grant and build "social credit." Here, we realize that an issue is far more important to the other party than it is to us. If we yield, we gain unspoken but understood favor with the other party.

Drawing from strong evidence regarding interpersonal tendencies for reciprocation, we give the other party what they desire with hopes that they will provide similar support on an issue that is important to us. The dance of interpersonal reciprocation and social credit is one that every effective negotiator has learned.

Pragmatically, postponing makes sense for two reasons. First, we should postpone when the emotional intensity is so elevated that it would be unduly risky and imprudent to try to move forward, at least right now. We realize that a calming period is needed. Second, we postpone when it is clear that we are less prepared than the other party. We need time to gather data and engage in reflection and study.[20]

The Respectful Conflict Encounter

Some conflicts must be addressed. The interpersonal and organizational impact of avoidance is too costly. Issues are recurring and are increasing dysfunction each time they arise. People are being affected either by direct conflict dynamics or increased tension because of unaddressed and unresolved issues. In short, the situation begs for action and the respectful conflict encounter approach is the preferred behavior. As a leader, your use of the respectful conflict encounter models expectations for others and establishes an interactive tone that will touch all aspects of culture.

The respectful conflict encounter is designed to be a one-on-one, eyeball-to-eyeball exchange. You work in a world of expediency where electronic data exchanges and remote connectivity prevail. They enable you to function, do your work and still have a life away from work. Tempting as it may be, these are not the mechanisms of respectful conflict encounter.

The argument, and we hear it all the time from physicians, is that it is next to impossible to blend schedules for a direct exchange. Yet we remain adamant. Unless prevented by unmanageable geographic dispersion, conflicting parties need to meet in person. These encounters are nuanced. Too many critical signals are lost when we veer from a personal exchange, and the risk of misunderstanding is simply too high.

Emotional Awareness and Regulation

We have addressed the elements of emotional intelligence in an earlier chapter. Here, we circle back and underscore the importance of these themes within a model of a respectful conflict encounter. Recall that we defined emotional self-awareness as the ability to recognize and understand our emotions, understand what caused them and realize how these feelings affect our thinking and subsequent behaviors. Researchers agree that emotional self-awareness is pivotal for subsequent regulation of those emotions.[21]

Issues of emotion regulation and self-regulation have received substantial and impressive research consideration.[22] We have noted some of the themes of emotion regulation already in this chapter. Here, we push beyond theory and consider application.

Impulse control — refraining from lashing out in an emotional fury — is a daunting challenge. Not only are we affected and aroused, but the other party is likely to exacerbate our arousal as the conversation unfolds. Consider an example, this time with the tables turned a bit. Lisa Brown is an administrator who needed to have a conflict encounter with Steven Mason, MD, a member of her team. She admitted that she was "somewhat intimidated" by Mason because of his status as the clinician expert on the team and his aggressive interpersonal manner.

Planning for the encounter, we asked Brown how Mason would likely respond when she presented her facts and why she felt the need to propose a direction that Mason did not want. "Oh, he'll be passive-aggressive. He'll flip his head dismissively and roll his eyes." Then she added, "I can feel my blood pressure spiking already. That makes me so mad."

Our advice was direct and certainly not earth-shattering. "Don't take the bait. Stay with the facts and the rationale. Then ask for his opinions."

Second, there are usually alternative ways to address issues that move the discussion ahead without letting it get emotionally overladen. For example, physicians have consistently complained to us about the glacial pace and wasted time that seems to be characteristic of so many meetings that they must attend as leaders. Frustration builds as issues are discussed ad nauseam and our minds wander to our busy agendas that are falling farther and farther behind.

As the emotional intensity builds, the tendency to express the obvious grows. "Damn, we're wasting time talking this to death." The veracity of this comment notwithstanding, others are likely to feel an affront and may believe that their views are being minimized or dismissed.

Here, we encourage an alternative approach — using the techniques of "summarization" and "forwarding the action." "As I've listened to the discussion, three themes seem to be recurring. First, our current nursing staff is feeling the pinch of salary compression. Second, we all agree that this needs to be addressed or we will experience unwanted turnover. Third, we are unlikely to have the funds to address these needs in the next year. Perhaps, since we agree on these points and constraints, we can move ahead and consider creative ways to address the issue in the next year."

Another technique for aiding impulse control is that of "filtered diversion." Let's return to our meeting example above. Filtered diversion encourages members to write down their feelings and thoughts before expressing them. As such, instead of saying everything we think, we have a safety valve. Two things occur. First, you gain time to think through the impact of what you are about to say. Second, once you see it in writing, you may recognize how imprudent the comments actually would be. Filtered diversion is most effective when it is applied generally as the first cues of frustration appear.

We present these themes up front before diving into the systematic conflict encounter process because emotional awareness and regulation will be needed throughout the process. Remember, even in the best process, the other party will not sit by idly, nod in agreement and readily acquiesce to your points and needs. Rather, we will get pushback, our emotional buttons will be pushed and our well-tempered emotional leveling will be challenged. That being said, let's move ahead.

The Desired Outcome

As a leader who is initiating a respectful conflict encounter, you must carefully define, in your own mind, your desired outcome. As basic as this seems, many people blunder into conflict without carefully defined outcome goals, and as such meander through an exchange that is probably too lengthy and too confusing.

In selecting an outcome of focus, do not aim for too much. The encounter is not the time to unload all issues and perceived transgressions of the past five years. Rather, be issue- and outcome-specific.

The Tone of Respect

The importance of respect has been discussed in an earlier chapter, as have the competencies of listening, expansive inquiry and dialogue. These considerations take center stage during conflict encounters. The key to any conflict encounter is to express your needs, your reasoning and your desires to another party, in short, to say what needs to be said. However, you must do so in a manner that maintains the self-respect and significance of the other party. Indeed, nothing prompts the other party's fight or flight syndrome more rapidly or dramatically than one's perception of being diminished, made less significant or being chastised in a disrespectful manner.

As in many situations, respect is signaled initially by your opening — your point of entry. It may be important to slow your pace of delivery. Some authors have even noted that it can be important to extend vulnerability by "leading with the heart."[23] You need not be over-the-top.

"I've been thinking about this for quite a while, and I feel we need to talk about our team meetings" can be a meaningful lead-in. Even this fairly innocuous start sends key messages of respect. For example, you signal the importance of the issue and by implication, the importance of the other party by noting that the encounter has been preceded by careful reflection. Further, you let the other party know that there is a large and important issue at stake — the team. It will appear that this encounter is prompted by broader team concerns rather than personal vendettas.

The Context and the Facts

As you begin the encounter, you need to explain the context — the specific situation you would like to address with the other party. We need to offer enough detail that both parties know the situation and events that are being considered.

As the initiator, you should check critical facts with the other party at this point. The inclusion of additional facts, especially those held by the other party, should provide greater clarity. This opportunity for all parties to put their facts on the table may help reframe the conflict or even eliminate the conflict entirely.

Stephen Covey illustrated this beautifully in his classic work *The 7 Habits of Highly Effective People.*[24] He tells of riding a crowded subway and experiencing deepening anger as a father sits idly by as his children bother other passengers. Unable to contain himself, Covey approaches the father and asks if he is aware that his kids are being a nuisance. The father apologizes and admits that he was not aware of his children's actions. Then, the father adds a previously unknown fact. We got on at the last stop — the hospital stop. Their mother and my wife just died and I guess we are not handling it well. Think back to the example of Hardy and her dean. I wonder what additional facts may have affected the dean's decision — some of which he may not have been able to share.

The Behavior

Once the context has been set and the facts have been clarified, you are ready to engage the heart of the conflict encounter. We begin by focusing on the specific behaviors or actions that are blocking the attainment of your expectations. It is critical that we emphasize behavior rather than inject assumptions about the other party's motivations, personality or character. Framing your comments by focusing on observable behavior rather than presumed intentions sets a tone of respect and helps move the conversation beyond personalities.

There is a subtlety here, but its impact can be dramatic. "I want to discuss why you went to the board with this issue" carries a far different impact from "I want to talk about the decision to take this issue to the board." The first is personal and will likely be perceived as accusatory. The second, hopefully, will be received more objectively, as a problem that needs to be solved. There is an additional advantage here. By emphasizing behavior, you are likely to be able to deflect emotional escalation for you and the other party.

The Impact

Statements of impact are idiosyncratic, drawn from your perceptions, impressions and assessments. Statements of impact are linked to the target behaviors, and take two forms: statements of personal impact and statements of "big picture" impact.

Statements of personal impact represent how the target behavior affects you on a personal and emotional level. While such statements may have limited sway with the other party, their candid expression does two things. First, it alerts the other party to how the behavior and resulting conflict are affecting you. This open expression suggests vulnerability and signals to the other party that you are aware of the personal dimensions of this conflict. Second, this statement gives you the chance to label your feelings and emotions rather than let others draw impressions that may or not be accurate.

As a rule, we favor labeling our own emotions instead of letting others place labels that carry the weight of personal agendas. It is better to say "I am disappointed and frustrated by this decision" than to have another implore me not to "get mad or angry." I do not want the "mad and angry" label when the appropriate label is really "disappointed and frustrated."

Statements of "big picture impact" are difference-makers. This is where you provide your impressions of what is at stake and how all parties are being affected. Motivationally, people are primed to behave in a manner consistent with their self-interests. Accordingly, if we can help another party understand how the target behavior negatively affects them and what they are trying to accomplish, your chances for impact are enhanced.

It is important to present the big picture impact for what it is — your impression of the big picture. Others may disagree. However, seek clarity to be sure that your view has been heard and understood. Pace down, clarify and assure the view is being received before moving on. Remember that your message of big picture impact, obvious and crystal clear, will be shaded and interpreted by others. Once again, we seek understanding and legitimatization, not necessarily immediate agreement.

Preferred Actions

In this step, you state what you would like to see happen — the preferred actions or behaviors that you seek from the encounter and exchange taking place. This is not the place for equivocation. Leaders should have clear prescriptive remedies.

Dialogue and Closure

As a leader and initiator of the conflict encounter, it is now time to invite the other party to share their impressions, needs and preferences. In short, you are requesting or extending an intention to dialogue. Hopefully, as you have modeled an open and respectful process, the other party will follow suit. However, as we have discussed in a previous chapter, dialogue is a process of nuance and finesse. Be sure to seek a full understanding of the other party's perspective and offer legitimacy of their view.

It is impossible and oversimplistic to become too formulaic at this step, but some caveats are appropriate. If and when the other party digresses and moves off-point, return to the target behavior. Briefly restate the big picture impact and your desired alternative steps.

Closing the encounter is a skill unto itself. Summarize what has been concluded, what actions will follow, who will be accountable and when the desired action will take place. It need not be overly extensive.

Focus and Wandering

There is a final caveat regarding the respectful conflict encounter. Stay focused on the issue at hand. The other party may attempt to cloud the conversation by wandering from topic to topic. In some cases, this is a deliberate deflecting strategy. In other cases, it is a means to save face. It may even be the product of an agitated mind, searching for common ground.

In any case, the appropriate response is to listen and acknowledge but bring the discussion back to the central issue at hand. "I understand that there has been a lot of pressure recently as we restructure. However, let's focus on the decision to get the director involved."

Out of the Blue

In the preceding sections, we described the respectful conflict encounter. This exchange is unique in that it presumes that we have time for planning and deliberation. In fact, we argued that difficult encounters should be approached carefully, the culmination of thoughtful reflection.

Realistically, we face many situations where we do not have the luxury of time, blunting our opportunities for in-depth analysis and gauged response. In many cases, conflict seems to arise spontaneously and unexpectedly.

Regardless of the likely array of precursors, we are either unaware of their content or surprised when they flare forward during a discussion or a meeting.

"Everything seemed to be going along nicely when out of the blue he became quite irritated and things got heated and personal." We want to address this inevitable situation and offer some perspectives that may be helpful. It sounds trite to say that the leader's true colors shine forth in the spontaneity of these encounters, but that will be the impression of those sitting around the table.

Leadership in the Face of Tension

We have already discussed, and you certainly understand, the complex array of behavioral processes that unfold. Yet, in the midst of the fray, understanding and enacting are often disconnected. Self-interest, ego protection and a range of emotions are activated as a member of the team touches a personal "hot spot."

Much like families, as teams interact over time, members learn one another's sensitivities and may purposely attempt to "push your buttons" to deflect discussion or to derail the pattern of action that is emerging. We have probably all experienced something resembling the following: "He never misses an opportunity to take a shot, to let us know we are intellectually inferior and to assert with undeniable certainty the truth of his views and the utter folly of ours."

Many of us take the bait, respond defiantly and escalate the emotional tone of the meeting. Admittedly, there are times when reciprocated assertion is necessary, especially when value issues or personal reputations are at stake. Leaders should not shirk these blatant calls for action. However, even in the depths of emotional upheaval, leaders must move judiciously to generate understanding and create opportunities for development and growth.

"Demands come from unmet needs."[25] It is one of the most succinct, pragmatic and conceptually accurate statements in the entire literature on conflict and negotiation skills. The corollary statement, which we have cited previously, is "Help me understand." These statements form a powerful frame of reference.

When encountering defiant blocking behavior, we should attempt to move from emotional arousal to conceptual understanding. Leaders begin by unpacking the event. What's going on? What prompted that? What is the unmet need? What's the understory? As such, our listening sensitivities and our skills of expansive inquiry must be engaged. "Help me understand why you want to go in that direction." "Help me understand why you feel this action represents a threat to your department."

We believe that if we probe deeply enough, a glimpse of the other party's logic will emerge. You may not agree. However, you can offer statements of understanding and legitimization. "So, if I'm hearing you correctly, you are concerned that this action will result in fewer resources for your department. Is that right? I can understand why that is an important concern."

Again, this ability to seek understanding and provide legitimacy of impact sets a tone of cooperation, collaboration and fairness (justice). It asserts that every view will be given consideration, even those that are offered in an angry, belligerent, aggressive or otherwise clumsy manner. Further, it demonstrates that you, as the leader, will unravel the insights and potential that are in the room, even among those who many of us would prefer to exclude. Your actions here will be a defining statement of your leadership.

We have noted that these skills may be a stretch for decisive, action-oriented, cut-to-the-chase clinicians. Recently, we sat in on a meeting led by a senior physician. He presented an issue (an undesired outcome) and asked the group members why they thought it had occurred. The first response came from a junior member of the team who offered her perspective. The leader, matter-of-factly, looked at her and stated, "No, that can't be what you think." There was a moment of chilly silence and then the room erupted into laughter.

Corrective Actions: Addressing Difficult People

At times, leaders are called upon to deal with difficult or problem people. While many of us might prefer not to do so, we must venture into this territory when any of three concerns are present: performance outcomes are threatened; others believe that inaction implies tacit acceptance and therefore smacks of inequitable treatment and injustice, and/or your leadership credibility will be undermined by inactivity.

In general, we avoid such encounters for three reasons. First, we do not cherish entering the encounter, which may be emotional and potentially explosive. Our reticence may be born of the sense that "let's not make things worse." This perspective is understandable but insufficient. Second, some avoid the encounter because they convince themselves that difficult people, obviously aware of their own deficiencies, will logically self-correct. This deluded thinking is inconsistent with what we know of the behavioral patterns of difficult and problem people. In many cases, they have convinced themselves that "everyone else is out of step." Third, and perhaps most striking, we avoid them because we are unsure of how to handle such encounters. Beyond these points, in most cases, some level of encounter is needed to prompt change.

There are two causal dimensions along which difficult and problem people may be viewed. The first is performance-related, where one performs below expectation. The second is behaviorally related, where one demonstrates behaviors that are interpersonally inappropriate or unacceptable. In short, these people just do not work and play well with others.

Realistically, when performance is dramatically below expectation, we act. By the same token, when behaviors are so caustic that performance and morale are destroyed, we respond. However, the rub for leaders is that difficult people rarely present at these extremes and mitigating factors are often present. Two categories of difficult or problem people are noteworthy: the "charming but unreliable" employee and the "talented but abrasive" employee.[26]

Charming but unreliable people are generally well liked. They have engaging and charismatic personalities and strong interpersonal skills. Their performance is not horrid, but it is sporadic and falls slightly below desired performance expectations. They may miss deadlines, turn in work that is below quality standards, miss some meetings, fail to get reports done on time or provide limited team contributions. Understandably, leaders can be reluctant to address these people precisely because of their warmth and likability. The leader's refrain goes something like this: "He's not the best we have, but everybody likes him."

The insidious issue here is one of perceived equity and justice. Others are "covering" for the charming but unreliable employee and "picking up the slack." Eventually, there will be a point of pushback and resentment where peers rail against what they rightfully see as a "special case." Despite our hesitancy, addressing the problem person before resentment manifests is the best course of action.

The "talented but abrasive" person is even more problematic. These people are skilled experts who bring an array of talents to their work. Often, they are technical or clinical experts in their respective fields. In addition, their performance reaches the highest standards. The concern is certainly not with performance but the interpersonal destruction that accompanies that performance. They tend to be adamant and inflexible. They are impatient and dismissive of others. They have little regard and tolerance for those who grasp issues more slowly than they do. They can be aggressive, demeaning, arrogant and hostile toward others.

The leader faces a dilemma, as the talented but abrasive person is both high performing and interpersonally destructive. They are among the elite experts in their fields. If they withhold performance, valuable outcomes are at risk. Further, their talents are not easily replaced. In the language of power politics, they rule the dependency game because we need their skills, skills that cannot easily be replaced. Consequently, fearful of ruffling the expert's feathers, many leaders choose to do nothing directly with the talented but abrasive person. In some cases, leaders even provide subtle reinforcement by encouraging others' tolerance. "Don't take it personally; that's just the way he is."

Unabated, talented but abrasive people can be toxic. They diminish morale. Others blanch when having to work with them. Positive cultural themes erode. And, as noted above, we will eventually reach a threshold of resentment as others question, "Why does she get away with this?" Failing to constructively respond, leadership credibility is threatened.

The model of respectful conflict encounters can be an appropriate guide for addressing problem people. Beyond this, we want to help problem people see the "gap" between performance and behavioral expectations and the actual outcomes and behaviors that they are exhibiting. We do this by carefully clarifying expectations and offering evidence to describe the gap. Our hope is that the difficult person will see the gap and feel compelled to close the gap. Actually, if we get to this point, working collaboratively to create a remedial plan of action will be the easy part.

Getting the difficult person to accept the gap is the trick. Often, these individuals are masters of excuses and emotion — both used to deflect attention from the gap. Rather than arguing over the veracity of given excuses or falling into an emotional tug-of-war, we suggest another action. When excuses and emotions arise; listen respectfully and return to the expectations. The expectations and subsequent gaps in expectations are the key issues to be addressed. When others use deflecting strategies, return to expectations.

This is a challenging conversation. Incremental progress can be expected. Further, problem people are notorious backsliders. They will improve for a while but soon slip back into some of their old patterns. Don't capitulate. Another conversation is needed. Incremental progress is still progress.

Concluding Thoughts: Organizational Bullies

There is a rapidly emerging area of behavioral research that addresses a growing problem — the presence of organizational bullies.[27] In some cases, bullies display such discriminatory actions that moral and legal demands necessitate strong disciplinary actions that may include dismissal. Most bullying behaviors do not rise to that level, but the bully's behaviors are often callous, dismissive, rude, intimidating, manipulative and disruptive. Unfortunately, in many cases, these behaviors are tolerated, especially when the bully has considerable expertise and skill that is not easily replaced. Such individuals fall into a category of problem people that have been labeled "talented but abrasive."[28] Interestingly, the line between abrasive and abusive is generally in the eye of the target victim.

When you are convinced that bullying is occurring, we suggest two actions. First, as the leader, you may need to have a conflict encounter to address the issues. Remember to focus on behavior and impact. Second, a "code of interpersonal civility" may need to be enacted. This clarifies for everyone certain words, phrases and actions that are "out of bounds."

---

1. Bohmer, R. (2012). *The Instrumental Value of Medical Leadership: Engaging doctors in improving services.* London: The King's Fund.

2. Ibid., p. 17.

3. Drucker, P.F. (2006). *Innovation and Entrepreneurship.* New York: Harper.

4. Jehn, K.A. & Mannix, E.A. (2001). The dynamic nature of conflict: A longitudinal study of intergroup conflict and group performance. *Academy of Management Journal, 44*(2), 238-251.

5. Schein, E.H. (2010). *Organizational Culture and Leadership* (4th ed.). San Francisco: Jossey-Bass, p. 301.

6. Ibid., p. 301.

7. Chen, M.J. & Ayoka, O.B. (2011). Conflict and trust: The mediating effects of emotional arousal and self-conscious emotions, *International Journal of Conflict Management, 23*(1), 19-56.

8.   Jandt, F.E. (1973). Conflict resolution through communication. New York: Harper & Row., p. 3.

9.   Jehn, K.A. & Mannix, E.A. (2001). The dynamic nature of conflict: A longitudinal study of intergroup conflict and group performance. *Academy of Management Journal,* 44(2), 238-251.

10. Boulding, K. (1962).

11. Stone, D.; Patton, B.; & Heen, S. (2010). *Difficult Conversations: How to discuss what matters most.* New York: Penguin.

12. Folberg, J. & Taylor, A. (1984). *Mediation: A comprehensive guide to resolving conflicts without litigation.* San Francisco: Jossey-Bass, p. 25.

13. Forsyth, D.R. (1990). *Group Dynamics* (2nd ed.). Pacific Grove, CA: Brooks/Cole.

14. Deutsch, M. (1973). The resolution of conflict: Constructive and destructive processes. New Have, CT: Yale University Press.

15. Nardone, G. & Watzlawick, P. (2005). *Brief Strategic Therapy: Philosophy, techniques, and research.* Lanthan, MD: Jason Aronson.

16. Mischel, W.; DeSmet, A.L.; & Kross, E. (2006). Self-regulation in the service of conflict resolution. In *The Handbook of Conflict Resolution: Theory and practice,* ed. M. Duetsch; Coleman, P.T.; & Marcus, E.C. San Francisco: Jossey-Bass.

17. Trenholm, S. & Jensen, A. (2013). *Interpersonal Communication* (7th ed.). New York: Oxford University Press, p. 117.

18. Metcalfe, J. & Mischel, W. (1999). A hot/cool-system analysis of delay of gratification dynamics of willpower. *Psychological Review, 106,* 3-19.

19. Baumeister, R.F. & Tierney, J. (2011). *Willpower: Rediscovering the greatest human strength.* New York: Penguin, p. 11.

20. Thomas, K.W. (1976). Conflict and conflict management. In M.D. Dunnette (ed.), *Handbook of Industrial and Organizational Psychology.* Chicago: Rand McNally, pp. 889-935.

21. Mayer, J. & Salovey, P. (1997). What is emotional intelligence? In P. Salovey & D. Sluyter (Eds.). *Emotional Development and Emotional Intelligence: Implications for educators* (pp. 3-31). New York: Cambridge University Press.

22. Mischel, W. (2014). *The marshmallow test: Mastering self-control.* New York: Hachette. Baumeiter & Tierney. (2011). *Willpower: Rediscovering the greatest human strength.*

23. Noer, D.M. (2009). *Healing the Wounds: Overcoming the trauma of layoffs and revitalizing downsized organizations.* San Francisco: Jossey-Bass.

24. Covey, S.R. (1989). The 7 habits of highly effective people: Powerful lessons in personal change. New York: Fireside.

25. Fisher, R.; Ury, W.L.; & Patton, B. (1991). *Getting to Yes: Negotiating agreement without giving in.* New York: Penguin, p.31.

26. Singh, K. (2007). *Counseling Skills for Managers.* New Delhi: Prentice-Hall of India Private Limited.

27. Bartlett II, J.E. & Bartlett, M. (2011). Workplace bullying: An integrative literature review. *Advances in Developing Human Resources, 13*(1), 69-84. Heames, J. & Harvey, M. (2006). Workplace bullying: A cross-level assessment. *Management Decision, 44*(9), 1214-1230. Saam, N.J. (2010). Interventions in workplace bullying: A multi-level approach. *European Journal of Work and Organizational Psychology, 19*(1), 51-75.

28. Singh, 2007.

7

Negotiations:
Influence and Principled Outcomes

A NEUROSURGEON HAS BEEN INTERVIEWING WITH SEVERAL FIRMS. He has had offers from three. One is his top pick. Despite this firm's eagerness to hire the talented neurosurgeon, the salary offered is $50,000 below the national average salary. As the neurosurgeon considers all the factors, he prepares to counter the firm's purposed salary.

An ER physician has to make the 2 a.m. call she hates to make. She has an elderly woman in her care with irregular heartbeats complaining of chest pains. Despite having a "normal" EKG, given the woman's age and history of heart problems, the patient needs to be admitted. But this woman's primary care physician is not one who enjoys being awakened in the middle of the night to admit patients. The ER physician dials the FP physician's number filled with anxiety as she braces for a heated discussion.

The director of a cardiac unit finished his presentation to the CEO, CFO and other key decision-makers at the hospital. He had outlined his need for additional funding to purchase new equipment that would bring the hospital to the cutting edge of cardiac technology. Despite liking the idea, the CFO stated that he had the money earmarked for another project.

All of the above situations are negotiations. Negotiations can be defined as "an interpersonal decision-making process necessary whenever we cannot achieve our objectives single-handedly."[1] From this perspective, negotiations occur whenever one person, in pursuit of specific goals, needs resources that another individual possesses. In a way, negotiations are much like conflict situations, in that both involve an interpersonal influence process. Often, conflict is the precipitating experience that activates the need to engage in negotiations.

Some negotiations seem incredibly straightforward — which restaurant to choose for lunch, which movie to watch or which hotel to choose. Others are complicated, involving multiple parties, complex terms and many conflicting needs. Yet one theme prevails. Whenever two or more parties must reach a joint decision but have differing needs, interests and goals, they negotiate.

All negotiations pivot on relationships, interactions and give-and-take exchanges. Fundamentally, all negotiations yield one of two outcomes: a negotiated agreement or an impasse. While a negotiated agreement is a preferred outcome, an impasse is not a sign of failure. Rather, an impasse signals that the parties are simply too far apart regarding their central needs to reach agreement at this time.

We can conceptualize many forms of negotiations. Of course there are contract negotiations, where parties attempt to agree on terms and conditions for the buying and selling of resources. This is the cinematic picture of negotiations, with businesspeople in suits sitting at large oak tables with lawyers, calculators and mounds of paperwork. The reality, though, is that most leaders rarely engage in this type of negotiation.

Instead, as leaders, we are frequently in negotiations with colleagues, supervisors, directors, staff and employees. We return to the basic definition of negotiations —"an interpersonal decision-making process necessary whenever we cannot achieve our objectives single-handedly."[2] Think about your work situation. Do you need the resources that another person possesses to accomplish your objectives? If so, you will negotiate.

At the root, negotiations are about obtaining necessary resources. From a leader's strategic point of view, resources may be composed of many forms and types. Perhaps you need more funding to hire a staff member. You have a need for a tangible resource — money. Perhaps you need public support from colleagues on an important decision. Here, you have a need for an intangible resource in the form of approval from important stakeholders. In both of these situations, you will need to influence another person to gain resources (money, approval and support) so that you will be able to pursue your goal.

In this book, we have focused on the interpersonal issues of leadership, and we will use the same focus for this chapter. We focus on the subtle interpersonal nuances that will help you be better negotiators.

At this juncture, an important point of distinction must be noted. Best-practice observations have indicated that most successful negotiators are not "in the moment" negotiators. Influential leaders understand that, in their work settings, negotiations occur regularly as strategic players within an organization vie for scarce resources.

At the same time, these same leaders realize that these negotiations will occur with individuals with whom they will have to interact frequently — perhaps even working together to pursue the same organizational goals. As such, the most successful leaders understand the social context within which negotiations take place. They realize that they need to focus on building social capital daily so that they are successful in negotiations. Rather than being "in the moment" negotiators, they become "constant" negotiators.

Constant negotiators grasp that negotiations are a process of interpersonal exchanges. They depend on and thrive on relationships. And, at their core, these negotiations are a process of influence. Further, they realize that influence does not happen at one point in time. Influence is an ongoing process that is embedded in social context and history. The constant negotiator works to build social capital and understands how to best influence other people. As such, we move our discussion to the research on influence within organizations.

Influence

Influence, or persuasion, can best be defined as "a change in the belief, attitude or behavior of a person (the target of influence) that results from the action of another person (an influencing agent)."[3] We conceptualize negotiations as a process that involves the use of influence tactics to persuade others.

In general, we classify influence tactics, or methods of influencing others, as being either "hard" or "soft." Hard tactics are those that use force or power to influence the other party. Commonly used hard tactics are legitimacy, pressure, exchange and coalitions.[4] Conversely, soft tactics are those that focus on subtly influencing the other party through psychological means. Commonly used soft tactics are rational persuasion, inspirational appeal, personal appeal, consultation and ingratiation.[5]

Hard Tactics

"Legitimacy" occurs when you remind the other party that you have formal power or authority — in essence the right to expect acceptance of your request. An example would be a manager reminding an employee that he or she will do something because the manager is the boss. The use of legitimacy implies the ability to use a pressure tactic.

The influence tactic of "pressure" relies on the use of warnings or threats. This is the proverbial hammer. An example would be threating a colleague to withhold needed resources if he does not act upon your request. Note that an individual can use pressure without having formal power, but formal positions of power, by definition, carry the ability to use pressure.

"Exchange" is more subtle, but it is still considered a hard tactic. With exchange, Party A is able to get Party B to do what Party A wants by offering Party B something desired. An example would be a leader asking an employee to work extra hours on a project in exchange for the leader championing the employee for a promotion.

Lastly, there is the use of "coalitions." By using the coalition tactic, Party A attempts to influence Party B by noting that other people (hopefully influential other people) feel that Party A's requests are appropriate and are supportive of the request. An example of a coalition would be group of followers trying to influence their immediate leader to decrease their level of work. The followers gain even more leverage when their coalition also includes staff members from unrelated areas and perhaps a key leader or two.

Hard tactics have their place in organizations, and they can certainly create influence. For instance, there are times when legitimacy and pressure are appropriate, especially when time is short and the risks are high. However, the research is clear: In general, hard tactics are not as effective as soft tactics.[6] In fact, the use of two soft tactics is often more effective than two hard influence tactics or a combination of soft and hard tactics.[7] Further, the use of some hard tactics, such as coalitions, tends to have a reverse (negative) effect on persuasion. For instance, we have often seen subordinates attempt to use a coalition with a supervisor, only to have the supervisor dig in his heels because he resents the notion of subordinates collectively talking behind his back.

Soft Tactics

"Rational persuasion" is a soft tactic where Party A uses logic and reason to explain to Party B why Party A's request is the best course of action. Another soft tactic is "inspirational appeal," when Party A explains to Party

B why a request helps reach a higher purpose or goal — in essence, appealing to some noble cause. Similarly, "personal appeal" occurs when Party A presents his request to Party B as a personal favor.

"Consultation" is also an effective soft tactic. In consultation, Party A asks Party B what is the best course of action, and during the ensuing open dialogue, Party A plants the original request in the mind of Party B so that it appears that the two have mutually developed the course of action.[8] This is particularly powerful, largely because it plays on the psychological aspect of "asking" people their opinion. In most cases, if individuals feel like they are being listened to, they are more likely to accept the decision, even when the final decision is not made in their favor. We return to the concept of legitimate voice — people feel like their opinions, concerns and views were considered in the decision-making process.[9]

Last, "ingratiation" is the use of pleasantries by Party A to try to build a liking by Party B. What is interesting about ingratiation is that individuals often have a negative reaction to this influence tactic if the true motive of the pleasantries is perceived to be an influence tactic. Thus, individuals who are high in political skill are better at using this tactic.[10]

Let's pull this all together and draw a few generalities. The research on influence in organizations has shown that the most effective tactics are rational persuasion, followed by inspirational appeals and then consultation.[11] The least effective influence tactics are pressure, legitimacy and coalitions.[12] This is important, and we will revisit these tactics as we dig more deeply into negotiations later in the chapter.

Combining of Influence Tactics

Of course, we do not just use one influence tactic at a time. Rather, we typically use a combination of tactics. In their research on influence and persuasion, David Kipnis and Stuart Schmidt noted four profiles of tactical combinations for "upward influence" — attempts to influence individuals with more power than the influencer. In their study, these researchers categorized the combination of influence tactics commonly used. Specifically, Kipnis and Schmidt noted that individuals used one of the following four combinations: shotgun approach, tactician, ingratiator or bystander.[13]

When attempting to influence others, individuals who use a shotgun approach used assertiveness, exchange and coalitions more than reason and ingratiation. Individuals who use a tactician combination rely on reason and exchange to influence others while relying less on ingratiation, assertiveness and coalitions. Individuals who use an ingratiatory combination use friendliness and exchange as their primary influence tactics. Finally, bystanders use relatively little of any of the influence tactics.[14]

In their work, Kipnis and Schmidt found that the least effective influencers were those who used the shotgun approach, and the most effective influencers were the tacticians.[15] In fact, tacticians had higher performance ratings, higher salaries and less job tension than individuals who used any of the other influence styles.[16]

Implications for Leaders

Let's highlight a few of the important findings. First, we know that the most effective influence tactic is rational persuasion. That is, individuals are best persuaded by arguments that are rooted in research and rational logic. To influence others, you must have a convincing story for why your request is the best course of action.

Second, we know that two other influence tactics are highly effective — inspirational appeals and consultation. In inspirational appeals, a leader attempts to influence others by showing how the leader's request actually plays into a much higher purpose or goal. The power of consultation occurs when it is used judiciously and with finesse. In using consultation, leaders meet with the person they want to influence, present the situation and ask the other person for suggestions for a solution. This begins a dialogue between the leader and the influencee in which the leader "subtly guides" the discussion so that the leader's original course of action is mutually developed and agreed upon.

Third, we know ingratiation is another tactic that can be useful but is potentially dangerous if done incorrectly. Ingratiation is the process of building likeability through the use of pleasantries. By "being nice" to others, the leader is attempting to "win over" the other party. We are more likely to accept requests of others whom we like than those whom we do not like. What is interesting about ingratiation is that it only works when the influencee does not know the true motive of the pleasantries. If influencees perceive there is an attempt to "kiss up," in most cases the effort will boomerang. Here, influence can be lost, trust may be damaged and foundations of relationships between parties may be diminished.

Fourth, we know from the research that individuals use combinations of tactics. And the most influential individuals in the workplace use a "tactician" approach, where they use reason and exchange much more than coalitions and assertiveness.

The Constant Negotiator

Taking these points together, we begin to see the tapestry in which the "constant" negotiator operates. Negotiating is building a context of style and an approach to relationships. This context is built over time. It precedes and continues beyond any direct and focused negotiating exchange.

Let's consider a few key points. First, constant negotiators realize that likeability and social capital are important during negotiations. They focus daily on building social capital by fostering and maintaining positive interpersonal dynamics, such as those that we have addressed throughout this book. They are pleasant and respectful during good times and hard times. Because of the consistency of behavior, their actions appear genuine. As such, these leaders have set the stage for being able to have discussions with others when they need to use influence tactics such as consultation. These leaders realize that it is hard to have the "let's think about a solution together" conversation if they have never shared a pleasant interaction with the other party.

It is easy to extend positive interpersonal exchanges and sensitivities to influential colleagues and other leaders, especially those with status and rank. Yet what of those people who seemingly have nothing to offer the leader? Why would a leader spend precious time asking a volunteer at the information desk about her day when there is nothing to be gained? This becomes a matter of character and tone.

Every small pleasant interaction actually can lead to a gain by creating a perception that you are a respectful person who is considerate of others. If your actions are directed only at a select few, when you need something, your true intentions may be questioned. Perceptions of manipulation probably loom in the minds of others.

Second, constant negotiators realize that they must be very logical when they are making requests of others. Thus, they gather information about important issues in an ongoing manner. They attempt to learn about the important aspects of negotiation issues from multiple stakeholders' perspectives so that they have a logical argument for all of those involved.

Succeeding Through Negotiations

Successful negotiators understand that negotiations are a process of influence. In the following sections we focus on how to prepare and engage in negotiations. We have drawn from a board range of research on negotiations and influence to give you better chance of succeeding during negotiations.[17]

Defining Your Success

How will you know if you have had a successful negotiation? Leaders need to start with the mindset that their "success" in a negotiation is when their goals are met. The first step to engaging in a negotiation is to determine your overarching goal. What needs are not being met? Consider what you are hoping to receive from the other party so that you are able to accomplish goals. What resource do they possess that you need?

As a leader, however, you need to think of goals in a broad conceptual sense. Your goals may focus on the greater good of the group you are leading. When you step into the leadership role, the question shifts from "what do I want?" to "what is needed to help me and my followers reach our vision?"

While setting the goals, you should focus on issues that are part of the language of negotiations. First, you must determine your "aspiration point" or "target point." This is your best-case scenario. In simplest terms, this is where you prefer or hope the negotiation will finally end. This goal must be salient in the negotiator's mind while engaging in the negotiation.

Second, you should also set your "resistance point." This is the point where the negotiator is ready to walk out of the negotiation. In fact, the term "walk line" is still used in collective bargaining contexts. This is the point beyond which you are simply unwilling or unable to go.

To determine the resistance point, we suggest that negotiators realistically assess their "Best Alternative to a Negotiated Agreement (BATNA)."[18] That is, negotiators consider the next best option if the current negotiating encounter reaches an impasse rather than a negotiated agreement. BATNA becomes your fallback strategy. A keen and constant awareness of your BATNA helps assure that you do not settle for an offer that will put you in a worse position than that available through your BATNA.

Let's consider a personally and admittedly simplistic example. A few years ago, I (the senior author) decided to replace my wife's original (and quite small) diamond wedding ring with a larger one — at least a full carat. After some shopping, two rings at two jewelry shops rose to the top of my list. The first was wonderful but seemed too pricey at $10,000. The second was acceptable and not nearly as nice, but carried a more palatable price tag of $7,500. This second ring became my BATNA. Thinking as negotiators, we realize that these prices are really the aspiration points of the respective jewelers.

Entering the negotiation for the first ring, I worked with the shop's owner. Drawing from my recently established BATNA and my limited funds, I set $8,500 as my resistance point. In other words, if I was unable to work a deal for $8,500 or less, I would walk away and purchase the second ring.

Now, here is the difficult part. I must somehow estimate the shop owner's resistance point — the lowest level at which he is willing to sell me the ring. I studied mark-ups on diamonds and chatted with friends, made my best judgment and structured my opening bid and subsequent negotiations with this perception fixed in my mind.

Objectively, even though I did not know it for sure, the shop owner had a resistance point. Let's assume that he had determined that he would sell that ring for no less than $8,000.

You can begin to see the situation unfold. The shop owner's resistance point is $8,000, and mine is $8,500. In essence, this represents what is known as "the bargaining zone." No negotiated agreement can exist outside this zone. If the shop owner held firm and refused to sell for $8,500 or lower, I walk away. If I refuse to pay at least $8,000, he looks for another customer. You see the evolving dynamics that are present in each negotiating setting.

OK, since the suspense is overwhelming, I bought the ring for $8,500.

Types of Negotiations

Negotiators should assess whether the negotiation is one of "opportunity" or "necessity."[19] A negotiation of opportunity, as the name implies, arises because a potential opportunity can be realized. A negotiation of necessity, however, must take place for the business to keep operating as normal. For example, one of your best friends from residency moves to the same area as you and asks for a job at your practice. Because you have no immediate and pressing staffing needs, this is a negotiation of opportunity. The practice, after all, is growing and your friend is quite skilled.

Consider a second condition, however. Here, your firm is short-staffed and you need to hire another physician so that you do not lose patients. This is a negotiation of necessity.

It is important to engage in negotiations of necessity before engaging in negotiations of opportunity. If an opportunity presents itself, successful negotiators only pursue that opportunity after they have finished negotiations of necessity, and after they have earmarked negotiations of necessity that are on the near-term horizon.

The next distinction is foundational and critical. Negotiations can be categorized as either "distributive" or "integrative."[20] In distributive negotiations, there is usually a single issue at hand, and when one party wins the other party loses — in short, a zero-sum game. In fact, distributive negotiations are situations "in which the issues at stake involve fixed sums of goods or resources to be allocated among the negotiating parties."[21] In distributive negotiations, one party's needs will dominate the other.

Conversely, when there is an integrative negotiation (also popularly known as principled negotiation), there is more than one issue at hand, and based on individual's preferences, issues can be traded off.[22] The process is intended to allow all parties to feel that their most important needs are met, even if some concessions must be made. All parties can leave an integrative negotiation feeling some level of success.

In the workplace, most negotiations have elements of both integrative and distributive bargaining.[23] Interestingly, many business negotiations have the potential to have integrative outcomes. In other words, many business negotiations have more than one issue that is being negotiated at a time. Sometimes multiple issues are not easily identifiable, but usually with careful thought and through interactions with the other party we can reveal more than one issue. Further, integrative approaches are preferred when ongoing interactions will occur.

The classic example may help.[24] There are two sisters who want to use the only orange they have for different reasons. The first sister wants the orange to make a glass of orange juice. The second sister wants the orange to make an orange merengue pie. The distributive "fair" way to solve the negotiation is for the sisters to split the orange. The first sister makes half a glass of juice and the second sister makes a pie that is half its original size. But, if the sisters view the orange as two issues — the juice and the pulp/rind — then there is the potential for an integrative negotiation. The first sister only needs the juice while the second sister only needs the pulp and rind. By thinking and negotiating integratively, both can get what they want.

Check Yourself

Just as with conflict management, we all have a "style" that we are most likely to use during negotiations. The literature presents three negotiating styles.[25] The first is "individualistic." People with an individualistic style are motivated to maximize their own goal pursuit without regard (or very little regard) to what the other party obtains. Contrast this style with the "competitive" style — a subtle but important distinction. People who pursue a competitive style focus on maximizing their own goals *and* minimizing what the other party obtains. Finally, people who have a "cooperative" style focus on fairness and equity. They want to make sure that both parties leave the table with some perception of gain — some sense that their needs and interests have been addressed.

There is a myth that good negotiators should be overly tough in their stances.[26] Indeed, many people believe that they must adopt a competitive negotiating style to be a good negotiator. However, it is the individualistic negotiator who is most likely to reach an integrative outcome. This may seem a bit counterintuitive. However, here is what we find. Individualistic negotiators are able to recognize which of the issues at play are most important to them, and they selectively focus on succeeding on those issues. Further, they are willing and able to yield on issues that are not important to them in order to reach their goals. Of course, this is the key to reaching an integrative outcome in a negotiation.

Conversely, people with a competitive style not only want to win on issues that are important to them but on issues that are not important to them. This creates a negotiation situation where the other party becomes less likely to make concessions because they are being asked to concede on all issues. As a result, the competitive negotiator is not able to reach his own goals as the other party reciprocates with a blocking positional stance.

Given our behavioral focus, many of you may have predicted that the cooperating style would be preferred. However, evidence suggests that individuals who use a cooperative style tend to give up more readily on issues that are important to them while obtaining more on issues that are not as important to them.

Keys to Principled Negotiations

Based on the abundance of research in the area of integrative or principled negotiations, we suggest an eight-step process for engaging in successful negotiations.[27] These are the keys to what has been popularly known as "principled negotiation." Roger Fisher, William Ury and Bruce Patton have noted, "In short, principled negotiations are negotiations that are integrative in nature and focus on maximizing joint outcomes between the two parties."[28] Remember, as specified earlier, most business negotiations have elements of distributive and integrative bargaining.[29] The goal is to find integrative solutions while maximizing gains and negotiating on distributive issues.

Information Is King

Leaders who are successful negotiators do an abundance of work before engaging in a negotiation. In short, they do their homework. When they are presented with a situation where a negotiation needs to take place, they begin by seeking and absorbing as much information as they possibly can about the issues. They research the issues. They talk with stakeholders about the issues. They consider the various angles of the issues. And they do this while trying to suspend their preconceived notions about what is the correct solution.

By gaining as much information as possible, there is a two-fold objective. First, the negotiator is drilling at the true need for the negotiation and uncovering potential obstacles to reaching an integrative outcome. Often by doing so, they develop a potential solution to the issue.

Second, they are gaining information so they can later build a rational argument to support their preferences. As we have stated earlier, rational arguments are inherently legitimate and are powerful influencers.

Remember that the key to reaching an integrative outcome is to look for tradeoffs. But how does a negotiator recognize the potential for tradeoffs? Again, information is key, but this time it is information regarding the other party and the perspectives and needs they hold.

Build Trust

As with so many themes in this book, trust again becomes a central concept. Research has clearly shown that when there is trust between negotiating parties, there is a greater likelihood that an integrative outcome will be achieved.[30] Logically, this occurs because the parties are more likely to share their preferences on the various issues being negotiated. They are less guarded and cautious. As a result, both parties are more likely to recognize opportunities for tradeoffs — satisfying the needs of both parties. Not surprisingly, established trust between parties allows negotiations to proceed more openly and more quickly than when trust is absent or uncertain.[31] Every statement does not have to be subjected to the scrutiny of due diligence when a foundation of interpersonal trust exists.

Building trust swiftly during negotiations is difficult. We return to the benefits of ongoing positive relationships in the workplace. If you, as a leader, have treated others in the workplace with respect and significance, then the building blocks of trust have the necessary foundation.

Further, trust begets trust; and trust stems from vulnerability. To build trust during negotiations, you have to make the first move. Share information about your perceptions of the issues and perhaps your preferences on a few of the nonessential issues. In most cases, people will react to such sharing by sharing information about their preferences as well. Here, we will draw on the well-established principle of reciprocity.[32] If you share information, others are likely to reciprocate by sharing information.

We need to note a caveat here; trust can have negative repercussions in negotiations. During distributive negotiations, if we extend more trust than the other party (and thus share more openly), it usually leads to fewer gains during the negotiation.[33] One more key point — while revealing information, you should never reveal your BATNA.[34]

Your style and manner of questioning are also important. To reach an integrative outcome, you should ask diagnostic questions.[35] Diagnostic questions are designed to elicit information about the other party's overlying interests. We suggest asking questions such as "What are your perceptions of this situation?" "What solutions would you propose?" And, "Of the issues that we have identified, which are most important to you?" The other party might not initially be entirely forthcoming, but by asking the questions you are showing concern and signaling your intent to look for mutually beneficial solutions.

Finally, we suggest that you ask only questions that you would be willing to answer yourself. We regularly caution those who negotiate with senior administrators to never ask a question or make a request that they would be unwilling to honor if they were sitting in the administrator's chair. Finally, after the other party provides their answer, take time to summarize their answers to be sure that you understand their responses correctly.

An Emotionally Safe Environment

Negotiations tend to spike emotional arousal. By their very nature, negotiations arise when individual's needs are not being met. When needs are not being met or others threaten our pursuit of meeting our needs, we tend to be have an emotional response. As we have noted in other places in this book, when we have a strong emotional reaction, we are using a "hot system" of thinking. When we are using the hot system of thinking, we may be in a state where we are reacting to our situation rather than behaving with rational intent.[36]

Remember, the best way to create influence in a negotiation is with the use of logical and rational persuasion, so it is important that we do not let our emotions overtake us during negotiations.

The other party is going through a similar process of emotional escalation. Their needs are being threatened, too, and they react accordingly. To prevent a situation of emotional escalation where the two parties begin to fuel negative emotions leading to a position stance among the negotiators, you have to work on developing an emotionally safe environment. You want to create an environment during the negotiation where you allow the other party to emote, yet do not allow their displays of emotions to influence the tone of the negotiation.

Good leaders work on building an emotionally safe environment by focusing on their own emotions and the other party's. First, let the other party see that you are understanding and empathic. Good negotiators listen closely to the other party when they become emotional; they search for meaning and provide nonverbal cues that indicate that the leader is engaged in active listening. They know intuitively that emotion generally arises out of frustration — the frustration of unmet needs.[37] Good leaders validate the emotions of the other party without necessarily validating the justification for the emotion.

Second, good leaders use emotional intelligence to keep their emotions in check during negotiations. Successful leaders are aware of their own emotional states and are able to regulate their behavioral responses that stem from those emotions. When they feel like they are having an emotional reaction and perhaps are likely to behave impetuously (often irrationally), they are able to "hit the pause button." That is, they suggest a break in the negotiation to allow the negative emotions time to subside.

Last, to build an emotionally safe environment, good negotiators listen and try to understand the backstory of the emotions. There is always a backstory, the "more to the story" to which we might not be privy. Successful negotiators realize that seemingly irrational emotional reactions by the other party are often completely rational to the other party. Good leaders listen and ask questions to determine why the other party's "hot buttons" have been pushed.

The Other Party's Story

It is important to try to understand the negotiation from the other party's point of view. Try to determine what issues are important to the other party. When we focus on others' perspectives of the issues, we are more likely to identify where potential tradeoffs could occur. Further, we are able to better identify which offers they are likely to accept.

It is never easy to assess the other party's story — their true interests and needs. In part, this is because people tend to talk in terms of positions or demands rather than the more critical foundations of interests and needs. We need to push beyond the demands and attempt to uncover the underlying needs.[38] Generally demands, and especially harsh demands, are reflective of some deeper unmet interest that is being threatened.

When developing your rational argument, it is important to focus on which logical arguments would make the most rational sense to the other party. Focus on how your proposal will help the other party meet their needs. Often people reject a negotiated agreement because they see the offer on the table that has too many obstacles for them to be able to successfully meet their own needs. Consider what obstacles the other party may perceive and give suggestions on how you can help remove those obstacles.

There are additional points regarding assessing the other party.[39] As noted in our earlier ring example, you should try to assess their BATNA. This is done so that you can make offers that play off their BATNA. For example, one physician was able to negotiate a higher salary because he knew the position had been advertised for more than a year — essentially meaning the hospital really did not have a BATNA! Thus, he was comfortable asking for a higher salary than they were offering because he knew they did not have a credible alternative.

Be a Problem Solver

The key to reaching an integrative outcome is to take a problem-solving approach to the negotiation. That is, you need to approach the negotiation as an opportunity to develop new solutions rather than a competitive joust. Successful negotiators realize that personalities at the table often cloud the negotiation. They realize that potential solutions lie in the facts of the situation. So they focus on the situation. Further, they try to find outcomes that both parties can agree upon and attempt to work toward that outcome.

Finally, successful negotiators focus on bringing in additional resources when needed. Remember that negotiations are about obtaining scarce resources, so when additional resources can be brought into the negotiation, there is a great chance a win-win outcome can be achieved. If we conceptualize distributive bargaining as "slicing the pie," we see adding resources as making the pie larger so everyone involved obtains a larger slice. For example, if you and a colleague are vying against each other for limited research money, perhaps through a joint effort, the need to negotiate could be reduced by applying for government research grants. In doing so, you are bringing more resources to the table.

The Give-and-Take

In this section we offer ideas on how to engage in a negotiation to reach the best outcome. We first focus on integrative outcomes. Remember, integrative possibilities arise when the parties have different preferences on the issues. For instance, you may care a lot about salary and not so much about the health care. Your employer may care about the total compensation costs, and as such be indifferent if you choose a higher salary as long as it is coupled with a commensurate reduction in overall costs. It is possible that the employer can increase your salary while not increasing his total compensation costs. Both parties get what they want and are happy. This leads to an integrative outcome.

The key to making this happen is what is known as "logrolling." Logrolling involves trading off issues.[40] It happens when parties recognize that they have different preferences for different issues. Through logrolling both parties experience success on their most critical needs.

Leigh Thompson has offered a series of suggestions for increasing the probability of reaching an integrative outcome.[41] First, as noted earlier, there should be a commitment to share information (but not your BATNA) and an attempt to build trust with the other party.

Second, negotiators should try to unbundle issues, meaning they should try to separate all the issues at hand and then prioritize them. Determine what issues are of the highest importance, what issues are secondary importance and what issues are of little importance.

Third, based on that assessment, negotiators should rebundle issues so that they develop multiple package offerings that are of equal value to the negotiator. By offering the other party multiple package offerings, the negotiator can learn which issues are important to the other party by seeing which packages are attractive to the other side.

For example, suppose the CEO of your hospital asked you to lead a new high-profile project. She stated that she wanted the project to serve as the new industry standard of "cutting edge." Further, she stated she wants the project completed in two months. She also adds that, although you will be given a modest bonus for completing the project, your work on the project must not interfere with your normal daily job responsibilities.

As you assess the situation, you determine there are three main issues at play in this negotiation: the quality of the project; the time frame in which the project is completed; and the amount of time working on the project that will interfere with your normal daily job responsibilities. As you further assess the situation and your daily job demands, you determine that it would be nearly impossible to deliver on all three of the CEO's demands. Thus, you can repackage the issues to develop multiple packages.

First, you could suggest that you could complete the project while continuing your normal job duties, but to have the highest of quality, the project would realistically take nine months.

Second, you could suggest that you could complete the project to the highest of quality in the two-month time frame, but you would need to be released from your normal daily responsibilities until the project was completed.

Third, you could suggest that the project could be completed in the two-month time frame while you perform your normal daily responsibilities, and that although the quality of the project will still be good, it will not be of the highest quality.

By making these three package offerings to the CEO, you are allowing the CEO an opportunity to implicitly indicate which of the three issues is most important to her by which package is most/least appealing to her. For instance, if the CEO flatly rejects the third option, you know that quality is the issue that is most important to her.

Regardless of whether the negotiation is distributive or integrative, you want to have your initial offer in hand before entering the negotiation. Further, if you have properly prepared by doing your research (i.e., determining your BATNA and setting your aspiration point), you may want to make the first offer.[42] This may seem confusing, as it defies conventional (and often errant) views that one should never make the first move. Actually, there is a sound theoretical foundation behind our advice, and it is known as the "anchoring bias."[43] The anchoring bias states that negotiations generally circle the first number that was within the zone of potential agreement.[44] Thus, by making the first offer, you are able to anchor the negotiation in your favor by presenting a number that is closer to your aspiration point. If the other party makes the first offer, it may be prudent to present a relatively quick counteroffer. By doing so, you re-anchor the negotiation for the other party. Further, by providing a timely counteroffer, you are giving a clear signal that you are willing to negotiate.

Once you make your offer, enjoy the silence.[45] More than likely, after you make an offer, the other party will be silent for a period of time. There is a natural tendency to assume that silence in negotiations is the precursor to rejection. In reality, often the other party is silent because they are just considering the offer made. Those who violate this guidance are likely to counter their own original offer — all because the other party does not respond immediately.

In distributive bargaining, alternative tactics work well to ensure greater gain. Remember, in distributive bargaining, we are negotiating one issue; that means the two parties must determine how to "split the pie." At some point, most negotiations have some element of distributive bargaining to them.[46] Thompson suggests that negotiators gain more during distributive negotiations when they make a few small concessions in the beginning stages of the negotiation.[47] Further, negotiators should follow a quid pro quo approach to making concessions. In doing so, they only give up a little at a time, wait for the other party to reciprocate, then repeat. Successful negotiators generally do not offer the other party ranges, because they realize that the other party only hears the number that is closest to their aspiration point rather than a range.

There really is no way to predict or formulaically prescribe this "dance" that is the nitty-gritty of negotiation. So we offer a few final pointers. Work together. Explore ways (options or approaches) that create mutual "wins." Brainstorm. Yield on less important issues to gain "social credit" that can be used to secure more important issues. Be reasonable — outlandish, over-the-top demands thwart progress, destroy trust and signal your intention to compete rather than work collaboratively. Try to get something in return when concessions are made, even if it is only to gain the aforementioned social credit ("OK, I can see this is really important.") Remember that "take it or leave it" approaches make wonderful drama, and they at times secure immediate success. However, their baggage will always be a drag on subsequent negotiations. As such, they should either be avoided or viewed as a last resort.

A Clear and Soft Landing

As the negotiation proceeds, there comes a time when you have to decide if you should accept the offer on the table. If you have prepared well for the negotiation by conducting research, you should know if the offer on the table is a good offer. When you decide that you would like to accept the offer, you must assess if the other party is ready for closure. You should present your perceptions of the agreement to the other party by asking, "Would you agree to ..." Hopefully they will accept and you can move forward and implement the specifics of the agreement.

What do you do if they do not agree? Even more critical, what do you do when you realize that you and the other party are just too far apart to reach an agreement? We suggest that in these cases you need to end the negotiation while allowing the other party to "save face." To do this, you want to summarize the final offer of the other party. Then reiterate your position on the issues. It is important to tell the other party that it appears that your needs are just too different at this point to reach an agreement. It is important that during this closing conversation you do not blame the other party for not being able to reach an agreement, but rather focus on the incompatibility of your goals and needs. An impasse today may simply be the first step in another negotiation a little farther down the road.

Psychological Strategies

The work of Deepak Malhotra and Max Bazerman focused on how to increase the likelihood of another party accepting an offer based on the attractiveness of the offer.[48] Their work noted that a negotiator can change the position of his offer, making it more attractive to the other party, without ever changing the material nature of the offer. As such, they suggest a number of psychological negotiation strategies.

Malhotra and Bazerman noted that individuals are more likely to accept an offer that has two small gains than one large gain and are more likely to accept an offer that has one large loss rather than two smaller losses.[49] For example, the offer of a 5 percent increase in salary and 5 percent increase in health care coverage is more attractive, psychologically, to individuals than offering a 10 percent increase in compensation. Conversely, individuals are more likely to accept an offer of a 10 percent loss in compensation than a 5 percent loss in salary and a 5 percent loss in health care coverage.

Further, Malhotra and Bazerman noted that individuals are more likely to accept an offer if it is positioned as to what the other party has to lose if they don't accept.[50] For instance, telling patients that if they quit smoking they are going to live longer is not nearly as persuasive as telling patients that they are going to die prematurely if they do not quit smoking.

Individuals are also more likely to accept an offer when more time and resources are invested in the negotiation.[51] That is, often individuals do not realize the sunk cost of negotiating. If they have spent time and resources trying to reach an outcome, they feel like that time and those resources will be lost if they do not reach an outcome.

Finally, the authors remind us that negotiators who are perceived to have several offers from other parties are less likely to have aggressive tactics used against them.[52] That is, if a hospital perceives that you are interviewing for jobs with several hospitals, they are less likely to use aggressive positional negotiating tactics.

Concluding Thoughts: Organizational Politics

Organizational politics is a term that often conjures up negative feelings. Most of us think of a "good old boy" network with backroom handshakes that act as the true driving forces behind happenings within the organization. And, as you might expect, many people have negative reactions to organizational politics. The research has shown that negative perceptions of organizational politics is a driving factor in employees' intentions to leave an organization.[53]

Unfortunately, organizational politics are the reality of organizational life. But, as Henry Mintzberg (one of the greatest organizational theorists of all time) has noted, politics are necessary in large organizations just to allow things to get done.[54] We contend that there are "necessary politics" and there are "toxic politics." As a leader, you have stepped into a new arena, where, to be a successful leader, it will become critical to engage in "necessary politics" while minimizing engagement in "toxic politics."

We define "necessary politics" as the politics that are played in order to build social capital and to help better the organization. These are behaviors that skirt the ambiguous lines around organizational policies (without cross-ing the line on personal ethics) with the underlying goal of improving the organization as a whole.

Conversely, we define "toxic politics" as behaviors that clearly violate or-ganizational policy and/or ethical guidelines to reach self-serving goals. An example of "necessary politics" would be a physician personally calling and asking a CEO, as a friendly favor, to consider funding her new project that would help her unit add value to the hospital. An example of "toxic politics" would be, in that same conversation, the physician talking negatively about the work habits of the other physicians who have made competing proposals.

Once social capital is built (and this should be an ongoing process), successful leaders use their social capital sparingly. Consider the analogy of sitting at a poker table. You have a set amount of chips (your social capital). Statistically speaking, it is unlikely that you will win every hand that you are dealt, so you would lose your chips very quickly if you played every hand. Successful poker players assess their chip count and decide when it is best to put their chips at risk. As a leader, you have to be just as strategic with your social capital. You can only play so many hands, so you have to be strategic with your choice of when to cash in your chips.

Even if you are a seasoned leader, we strongly suggest you avoid engaging in "toxic politics." The problem is, playing these sorts of politics is tempting. We have all witnessed individuals in the workplace who get their way because they wield their political power and shape perceptions of others in their favor by feeding into the rumor mill. The gains that toxic politics bring are momentary and fleeting. Colleagues of "toxic politicians" begin to form resentments and coalitions against them begin to form. And in time, more often than not, those who overly rely on toxic politics eventually fall.

---

1. Thompson, L. (2004). The heart and mind of the negotiator. Upper Saddle, NJ: Pearson-Prentice Hall.

2. Ibid.

3. Raven, B. H. (2008). The bases of power and the power/interaction model of interpersonal influence. *Analyses of Social Issues and Public Policy, 8*(1), 1-22.

4. Falbe, C. M., & Yukl, G. (1992). Consequences for managers of using single influence tactics and combinations of tactics. *Academy of Management Journal, 35*(3), 638-652.

5. Ibid.

6. Ibid.

7. Fable & Yukl (1992); Higgins, C. A., Judge, T. A., & Ferris, G. R. (2003). Influence tactics and work outcomes: a meta-analysis. *Journal of Organizational Behavior, 24*(1), 89-106.

8. Yukl, G., & Falbe, C. M. (1990). Influence tactics and objectives in upward, downward, and lateral influence attempts. *Journal of Applied Psychology, 75*(2), 132-140.

9. Korsgaard, M. A., Schweiger, D. M., & Sapienza, H. J. (1995). Building commitment, attachment, and trust in strategic decision-making teams: The role of procedural justice. *Academy of Management Journal, 38*(1), 60-84.

10. Harris, K.J., Kacmar, K. M., Zivnuska, S., & Shaw, J. D. (2007). The impact of political skill on impression management effectiveness. *Journal of Applied Psychology, 92*(1), 278-285; Ferris, G.R.; Treadway, D.C.; Perrewé, P.L.; Brouer, R.L.; Douglas, C., & Lux, S. (2007). Political skill in organizations. *Journal of Management, 33*(3), 290-320.; Treadway, D.C.; Ferris, G.R.; Duke, A.B.; Adams, G.L., & Thatcher, J.B. (2007). The moderating role of subordinate political skill on supervisors' impressions of subordinate ingratiation and ratings of subordinate interpersonal facilitation. *Journal of Applied Psychology, 92*(3), 848-855.

11. Fable & Yukl (1992).

12. Ibid.

13. Kipnis, D., & Schmidt, S. M. (1988). Upward-influence styles: Relationship with performance evaluations, salary, and stress. *Administrative Science Quarterly*, 528-542.

14. Ibid.

15. Ibid.

16. Ibid.

17. Fisher, R., Ury, W., & Patton, B. (1991). Getting to yes: Negotiating agreement without giving in. New York, NY: Viking Penguin. Diamond, S. (2010). Getting more: How to negotiate to achieve your goals in the real world. New York, NY: Crown Business; Shell, G.R. (2006). Bargaining for advantage: Negotiating strategies for reasonable people. New York, NY: Penguin Group; Fisher, R. (1995). Getting ready to negotiate. New York, NY: Viking Penguin; Levinson, J., Smith, M., & Wilson, O. (1999) Guerrilla negotiating. Hoboken, NJ: Wiley; Kramer, H. (2001). Game, set, match: Winning the negotiations game. New York, NY: ALM Publishing.

18. Brett, J.F., Pinkley, R.L., & Jackofsky, E. F. (1996). Alternatives to having a BATNA in dyadic negotiation: The influence of goals, self-efficacy, and alternatives on negotiated outcomes. *International Journal of Conflict Management, 7*(2), 121-138.

19. Thompson (2004).

20. Walton, R.E., & McKersie, R.B. (1965). Behavioral theory of labor negotiations: An analysis of a social interaction system. New York, NY: McGraw-Hill. Lax, D.A., & Sebenius, J.K. (1986). The manager as negotiator: Bargaining for cooperation and competitive gain. New York, NY: Free Press; Kong, D.T., Dirks, K., & Ferrin, D. (2013). Interpersonal trust within negotiations: Meta-analytic evidence, critical contingencies, and directions for future research. *Academy of Management Journal*, amj-2012. 0461.

21. Barry, B., & Friedman, R.A. (1998). Bargainer characteristics in distributive and integrative negotiation. *Journal of Personality and Social Psychology, 74*(2), 345–359, p. 345.

22. Thompson (2004); Lax & Sebenius (1986).

23. Lax & Sebenius (1986).

24. https://cramaswamy.wordpress.com/2010/08/06/integrative-negotia-tion-%E2%80%93-tale-of-two-sisters-and-an-orange/ .

25. Thompson (2004).

26. Thompson (2004).

27. Fisher, Ury & Patton (1991); Diamond (2010); Shell (2006); Fisher (1995); Levinson, Smith & Wilson (1999); Kramer (2001).

28. Fisher, Ury & Patton (1991).

29. Lax & Sebenius (1986).

30. Kong, Dirks & Ferrin (2013).

31. Covey, S.M.R. (2006). *The Speed of Trust: The one thing that changes everything.* New York: Free Press.

32. Shell (2006).

33. Kong, Dirks, & Ferrin (2013).

34. Thompson (2004).

35. Thompson (2004).

36. Weiss, H.M., & Cropanzano, R. (1996). Affective events theory: A theoretical discussion of the structure, causes and consequences of affective experiences at work. In Staw, Barry M. (Ed); Cummings, L. L. (Ed), Research in *Organizational Behavior: An annual series of analytical essays and critical reviews,* Vol. 18. , (pp. 1-74). US: Elsevier Science/JAI Press.

37. Fisher, Ury & Patton (1991).

38. Ibid.

39. Thompson (2004).

40. Froman, L.A., & Cohen, M.D. (1970). Research reports. Compromise and logroll: Comparing the efficiency of two bargaining processes. *Behavioral Science, 15*(2), 180-183.

41. Thompson (2004).

42. Galinsky, A.D., & Mussweiler, T. (2001). First offers as anchors: the role of perspective-taking and negotiator focus. *Journal of Personality and Social Psychology, 81*(4), 657.

43. Bunn, D.W. (1975). Anchoring bias in the assessment of subjective probability. *Operational Research Quarterly,* 449-454.

44. Galinsky & Mussweiler (2001).

45. Thompson (2004).

46. Lax & Sebenius (1986).

47. Thompson (2004).

48. Malhotra, D., & Bazerman, M.H. (2008). Psychological influence in negotiation: An introduction long overdue. *Journal of Management.* 34(3): 509-531.

49. Ibid.

50. Ibid.

51. Ibid.

52. Ibid.

53. Cropanzano, R., Howes, J. C., Grandey, A.A., & Toth, P. (1997). The relationship of organizational politics and support to work behaviors, attitudes, and stress. *Journal of Organizational Behavior, 18*(2), 159-180.

54. Mintzberg, H. (1985). The organization as political arena. *Journal of Management Studies, 22*(2), 133-154.

8

Motivation:
Building Performance Through People

....

⫽⫽HOW DO I MOTIVATE MY PEOPLE TO HIGHER LEVELS OF PERFOR-
mance?" It is one of the most common questions we are asked when others
learn that we specialize in management and leadership. The answer is complex,
and no topic within our field has garnered more research attention.[1]

At one level, this research has helped us understand that performance
arises from the interaction of two factors — ability and motivation.[2] Through
proper hiring, placement and training, we can help ensure that our employees possess the ability to perform and we can design jobs so that employees
have the opportunity to perform. But the question of how to motivate is much
more complicated.

Motivation is a personal, internal decision, and even the best among us
are unable to "make" someone be motivated.[3] Yet we can affect motivation.
We can create conditions and contexts that promote motivation and enable
it to flourish. We can structure situations and take actions that help release
the potential of our people.

In this chapter, we will consider specific theories of motivation. In many
ways, it all comes down to one main factor: knowing your people. Leaders
who know their people — understanding what they care about, grasping
their career aspirations, and recognizing the scope of their abilities, talents,
strengths and weaknesses — are poised to positively affect motivation and
subsequent performance. It's an exciting journey, and we begin with a bit
of theory.

Need Theory Foundations

One of the earliest views of motivation was proposed by Sigmund Freud and is commonly known as the "pleasure principle."[4] Basically, Freud contended that individuals seek pleasure and avoid pain. If something provides an employee pleasure, she will increase behavior to gain it.

For example, if an employee enjoys interactions with others, she may frequently place herself in situations that allow her to engage others in conversation. Further, she may avoid or decrease behaviors that require isolation, such as balancing accounts in the deserted bookkeeping room. While overly simplistic, the pleasure principle is the foundation for much of our motivational thinking. However, we must recognize that not all people have the same pleasure states. In other words, people are motivated by different factors.

The conceptual foundation of need theories is that our needs (and the pursuit of our needs) influence motivation. Classic need theory stipulates that our needs are arranged in a predictable hierarchy of importance.[5] First, people strive to meet their physiological needs — those that are fundamental to existence. Once these needs are sufficiently met, we address our need for safety. Only after these basic needs are reasonably assured do we progress to the third level, of social needs. Self-esteem needs follow. Finally, the need of self-actualization will receive attention when the previous needs in the hierarchy have been met satisfactorily.

The hierarchy and many of its underlining hypotheses have been augmented through the years. We prefer E-R-G theory, a more recent need model. Rather than the classic five-tiered model, E-R-G postulates that individuals are working to meet three fundamental and successive needs: existence (physiological and safety needs); relatedness (social needs); and growth (self-esteem and self-actualization needs).[6]

We also find it helpful to conceptualize needs as higher order (relatedness, social, growth, self-esteem and self-actualization needs) and lower order needs (existence, physiological and safety needs).[7] Lower order needs are finite. Once we feel that we have a sufficient level (known as gratification), they no longer provide motivational impact. Higher order needs, however, are infinite in nature. Securing some level of these needs generally prompts the desire for more.

Let's consider the movie *Cast Away* to gain some context. Tom Hanks' character, Chuck Noland, becomes stranded on a deserted island. The movie is largely remembered because of Wilson, a volleyball, Noland's companion. When Noland was first stranded, his first actions were not to make friends with ocean debris. He was first motivated and driven to find a source of food to sustain life; he was motivated to make shelter and a fire to provide him with safety. Only after those needs were satisfactorily met did he start to be motivated by his lack of social interactions.

Need theories underscore at least two important themes. First, people behave (are motivated) to meet needs. Second, these needs will change as circumstances change.[8] Further, people work on multiple needs at once, and the need that is most salient can change relatively quickly. As such, a need that was predominant (and therefore the focus of motivation) at one time is likely to be replaced by another predominant need at a different time.

For example, a newly graduated doctor with significant educational debt may be primarily motivated by salary. Fast-forward 10 years, and that same individual is financially stable and may be more focused on establishing his practice and learning new skills. Fast- forward 10 more years, and that same physician may want to devote more of his time to a community clinic, assisting patients who live in poverty. Motivation for this physician has changed with his changing needs.

As a leader, it is useful to stay attuned to the shifting maze of employee needs. This requires time to talk with people, and most important, to listen. Asking questions to determine your employees' career goals may help in determining their needs, thereby providing a more accurate focus for your motivational efforts.

Understanding needs is important for understanding how to motivate others. However, as a leader, you must recognize that others may not be (and probably are not) working on the same needs as you. Enter projection, a concept that is given too little attention in leadership. Projection is the tendency to assume that other people have the same personality and motivations as ourselves.[9]

The consequences of projection can be dramatic. When we assume that other people have similar personalities to ours, we likely have lower tolerance for people who are less detail oriented, less conscientious and less driven to meet our lofty standards. When we assume that other people have similar motivations as ourselves, we fail to understand why working overtime "just because the project is so exciting and challenging" does not capture others' energies. Projection also applies to needs. We may assume that others are working on the same needs as we are. Awareness of projection is a cautionary theme for highly driven, inner-motivated leaders.

Themes of Physician Motivation

Highly trained, highly competent professionals offer unique motivational challenges. While you deal with a range of clinicians and staff personnel, the motivation of fellow physicians may create some of the more problematic issues you will face. Consider the following example, garnered from a physician interview.

Mike Jones is a board-certified emergency room doctor who works in a Level 2 trauma department. Jones has been practicing medicine for 10 years. As with many people, he loves his job, and he hates his job. We asked "what motivates you," and he provided an insightful explanation:

> "It's difficult to say, it changes at different points of my career, and it changes day to day, and environmental factors change my day-to-day motivation ... I guess at the heart of it is to take care of patients. That was the initial inspiration to practice medicine and still is today, but in a different respect. But on a day-to-day basis while I'm in the ER working, I'm pretty motivated to practice good medicine.
>
> "Despite health care being so messed up, despite the crap that I have to deal with in a difficult patient population, despite the stress of malpractice lawsuits, when I ask myself, "Why did I get into this?" it's to help patients. Really the only thing that makes it all worthwhile is that I am doing something good. I mean I really believe I am doing something good here — my patients are in crisis and I'm helping. You know, you are doing something good for society.
>
> "But you have to remind yourself of that. No one thanks you. I count the lives I've saved. I mean, I remember this one guy, he was dead ... he was flat lined, and I saved him.
>
> "But did he thank me? No. So it's a thankless job, with the stress of liability, and yeah, I'm getting paid enough, but at some point you have to look at what you do and the impact it has on humanity.
>
> "You know, one day I want to practice international medicine — for

free. I want to do that — provide a quality of care for people who can't af-
ford it or don't have the access like we do here — but I'm not in a position,
financially, to do that.

"I have to say I feel that anyone who tells you money is not a motivat-
ing factor is lying. But that's what I was saying about different motivators
at different times. Like when I get up in the morning after a few days off,
I don't wake up and say, 'Can't wait to go save lives!' No, I think, 'This is
going be another long day in hell, but I have to get into work so I can afford
to live.' But once I'm there, in the thick of it all, the money is definitely not
worth it, at that point I shift to thinking about saving lives."

What do you think? What is Jones' primary motivator? How does he see
that changing? What do you think would be motivating for him right now?
What motivational opportunities seem to exist?

Indeed, he is motivated by salary. However, he also desires recognition
— recognition that his work is significant and that he does a good job. In-
trinsically, he knows these things. Yet he seems to yearn for more external
validation. Of course, we cannot assume that his motivations are the same
as other physicians or others who work in the medical field. Jones' interview
reveals another recurrent theme about his regard for patient care. Not surprisingly, researchers have noted that "physicians are inherently motivated
by their desire to provide high-quality patient care."[10]

Overall, studies on physician motivations are rare.[11] However, research
examining work preferences for physician scientists has provided some
important perspectives.[12] Here, four main factors emerged: recognition,
compensation, the challenge of the work and the importance of the work. In
a similar vein, Michael Trisolini found that financial compensation, lifestyle,
recognition and patient appreciation were keys to physician motivation.[13]
Others found that feelings of accomplishment on difficult tasks, satisfaction
with clinical outcomes, autonomy, respect and collegial relationships were
primary motivators for physicians.[14]

Although these studies are by no means exhaustive, they do point to
some common themes. Yes, compensation is a factor. However, other factors
seem to be just as important in motivating physicians, if not more important.
The impact of the work being performed, the feeling of accomplishment for
completing a difficult and challenging task, recognition, autonomy and re-

spectful collegial interactions all seem to be keys.

We would be remiss if we did not acknowledge one other motivating factor for physicians — identity. Physicians have a certain level of status in society, and for some this plays an important part in their motivation to be a physician.

From Behavior Modification to Leadership

Our current views of behavior modification are derived from the classic work of B.F. Skinner. Most, if not all, compensation systems are designed to increase motivation, and the basis for these compensation systems is behavior modification. Drawing from the pleasure principle, we modify the behaviors people perform in the workplace by providing rewards they desire.

To change behavior or motivate performance, a five-step process known as behavior modification is useful.[15] The first step in behavior modification is to identify the behavior you want to change (or motivate). The second step is to measure the behavior you want to change before making any changes. This baseline measurement is important so that we can later assess whether our reward system is actually affecting the desired behavior.

During step three you will think about potential problems or unforeseen consequences that may arise. For instance, if we reward quantity, what are the implications for quality? The fourth step is to apply the reinforcement. (We will address this topic in more detail in the next section.) Finally, in step five, we re-measure the behavior to see if the desired change in behavior has occurred and then adjust as needed. Simple, right?

Well, not exactly. That is just an overall blueprint of how to motivate individuals in the workplace. This is the black and white of motivating. As we know, leadership often occurs in the gray — the real application of principles. Behavior modification in organizations is filled with nuances to which leaders must be attuned.

First, let's examine the various types of reinforcements that can be applied. Positive reinforcement provides individuals something they value as a means to increase the desired behavior. Negative reinforcement attempts to remove something that is noxious or unpleasant to increase a desired behavior. The goal in both of these types of reinforcement is to increase a desired behavior.

At this point we should talk about punishment. In punishment, the goal is to decrease an undesirable behavior. As such, no new learning occurs. Behavioralists generally shun punishment. Instead, the focus is on reinforcement — inspiring and trying to encourage positive, desired behavior. Further, research shows that overuse of punishment by managers can build resentment in their employees.[16]

For behavior modification to work, you must understand your people and their needs so that the reinforcement you apply helps meet relevant and salient needs. Perhaps you want one of your team members to work extra hours for the next month. How would you entice him do to so? Perhaps you'd offer extra pay. This may motivate a person who is concerned with making money. Perhaps instead you could offer extra time off at a future time. This reinforcement may be more motivating for an employee who is planning a vacation in the future.

Next, for behavior modification to be efficient, people must know what they are working toward. Leaders have to set clear expectations and explicitly state the link between meeting these expectations and receiving rewards. It is useful to provide a path to success so that people understand which behavior will be rewarded.

Let's examine the behavior modification model in action through an example. Let's say you have decided that your practice would be more profitable if you were able to see more patients. You notice that one of the "clogs" in your ability to see more patients is that your nurses are spending more time than is needed with each patient. In this manner, nurse efficiency — the amount of time each nurse spends with each patient — is the target behavior that you want to affect.

Next, you would gather baseline data — the amount of time each nurse is spending with each patient. Then you would attempt to anticipate any unwanted consequences that might result from your modification system. In this instance, is there a possibility that lowering the time each nurse spends with a patient could impair the amount of information the nurses are able to obtain from patients regarding their medical issues? Is there a possibility that lowering the nurse-patient contact time could lower overall patient satisfaction? Suppose you do this assessment and decide that the benefits of lowering nurse-patient contact time outweigh the potential negatives. You would proceed to the next step.

The next step would be to inform your nurses of the new behavior you will be rewarding and how you will be rewarding it. Let's say you decide that you are going to give a 1 percent paycheck bonus for nurses who were able to maintain a determined average nurse-patient contact time. Of course, you would adequately explain the reason behind the rewards and the desired behaviors. Finally, after applying the reinforcement, you would re-measure the contact time to see if the desired effect occurred.

Again, sounds simple, yet there are additional complexities. First, remember that not all people are working on the same needs — so money might not be the most powerful motivator for all individuals.

Another peculiarity of the behavior modification system pertains to cognitive evaluation theory.[17] Cognitive evaluation theory does not apply to all individuals, but it is something that should be considered. This theory argues that there is a risk of diminishing intrinsic motivation when an extrinsic reward is attached to a behavior that a person was performing of their own volition. That is, if a person is performing a behavior because they want to — an internal driver — the presence of a reward might diminish or even extinguish the internal drive to perform.

Sometimes this phenomenon happens when individuals are volunteering and then are offered a job doing the same thing for which they had previously volunteered. They perform the same behaviors, but they no longer find the same internal satisfaction in doing the behaviors or actions. The reason is the sense of control over the behavior has shifted from one's internal control to a sense of being "forced" to perform the behavior by external factors — in this case, pay.

Let us examine how cognitive evaluation theory might influence the use of the behavior modification system. One area where this can be an issue is with mentoring. Some individuals mentor new employees because they enjoy it and find the process fulfilling. As such, they take on a mentor role without any forethought of compensation. This is generally appreciated, as there are a host of benefits that come from having high-quality mentors in an organization. However, some organizations have attempted to formalize mentoring activities by offering bonuses or other rewards (release time from other duties) to encourage more people to become mentors. Essentially, these organizational leaders are applying a behavior modification system — attempting to increase mentoring by providing monetary reinforcement.

What will happen?

Assuming that the proper rewards are in place and your people understand what behaviors they are being rewarded for, mentoring should increase among all the followers. The followers who were previously not mentoring will start mentoring. This is the desired effect of behavior modification. The followers who were previously mentoring will likely continue mentoring.

But what happens to that latter group's intrinsic motivation? They may no longer possess the internal drive to do the behavior because they are now being told to do the behavior.

As long as you are able to continue the external reward, there should be no problem in installing such a behavior modification system. But, let's consider that the reward (perhaps for financial reasons) has to be withdrawn. What is the result? First, the group of followers who were performing the behavior solely for the reward will probably stop performing the behavior once the reward is removed. Second, the group of followers who were performing the mentoring behavior before the reward system was applied are unlikely to return to their original baseline. Again, mentoring activity is diminished. By attaching a reward to the behavior, the intrinsic motivation has been subverted.

Another issue that should be considered is the way that behavior modification systems may be limited in the medical field. For certain behaviors, there are standard practices of care. Thus, by rewarding those behaviors, medical professionals are unlikely to respond by increasing their behaviors. For instance, in a three-year study in at an oncology center, there was no increase in the number of cervical cancer tests as a result of rewarding physicians for the number of cervical cancer tests ordered — despite more than $100 million being allocated as incentives.[18] What this study shows is that on some issues, physicians will behave in accordance with standards of care and their behaviors largely will be unaffected by incentive systems.

A final note: Behavior modification systems work well for behaviors that are routine and relatively simple, where we can clearly specify behaviors that will lead to higher performance. However, the traditional behavior modification system does not work as well when individuals are working on non-routine tasks.[19]

For instance, if the goal is to increase creativity or problem solving, the traditional behavior modification systems are limited because they encourage individuals to focus on predetermined solutions. One study examining the effects of incentives on physician behavior found that physicians took specific actions to reduce the use of resources when they were rewarded for cost-reducing behaviors.[20] However, the problem solving of these physicians (and their teams) did not increase. In a field where the norm is the exception and most cases have their own specific issues, thus requiring problem solving, we need to make sure that behavior modification and incentive systems do not stifle the creative process.

Foundations of Equity

Rooted in the psychological research on social comparisons, equity theory helps us understand individual motivation and performance. Fundamentally, equity theory revolves around perceptions of fairness. If people believe that they are being treated fairly (and rewarded fairly), motivation and performance are positively affected. However, when people experience perceptions of unfair treatment with unfair outcomes, motivation wanes and performance may be diminished.[21]

As with any perception, the theory revolves around the ways in which people assess fairness. In short, most of us cognitively determine a simple ratio of the rewards that are received (such as salary, recognition or any factor that is valued) versus personal effort expended (time and energy). We then compare this ratio to our perception of the reward/effort ratio of others. These referent others are used for comparisons when judging fairness.

We conduct these social comparisons regularly. Consider the following example. Each year, as salary adjustments are announced, the process begins. The actual percentage of salary increase has tangible importance. However, its motivating potential is also tied to perceptions of equity. A 2 percent increase in salary may seem rather paltry, especially given the hard work and accomplishments you provided over the past year. But is it fair and equitable?

The perception of equity is derived from others. Were colleagues who contributed far less compensated at a commensurately lower rate? Think of the impact when you learn that your 2 percent increase was the highest rate in the entire system for this year. Think of what it means when you learn that only the top 1 percent received your level of increase. Consider the impact when you learn that a low-performing colleague received no increase. Motivation and willingness to expend future efforts likely have been positively affected.

While various categories of referent others exist, two are especially important: the "other-same" (comparing yourself to others who are in a similar position as you — usually colleagues in the same organization); and the "other-different" (comparing yourself to others in a different organization — usually professional colleagues). In clinical contexts, where the capacity for mobility is high, both categories are likely to be used for comparisons.

When we compare our reward/effort ratio to a referent other and perceive imbalance, we are motivated to address the inequity. In general, a series of actions are likely to take place. First and most common, we may reduce our effort. Second, we may seek greater rewards. Third, we may choose to exit the situation and take our talents elsewhere.

This theoretical view provides practical impact, especially in our highly competitive world. Sometimes individuals perceive inequity because they are comparing themselves to people who are not comparable and relevant referents. People also tend to cognitively distort their perceptions of their efforts — an "overvaluing bias." In addition, people often have inaccurate perceptions of the rewards that others receive, believing others receive attention, special consideration and additional benefits that are simply inaccurate.

As in so many areas, openness and communication are key. Of course, in some areas, especially those involving compensatory issues, we must exercise caution and restraint. Correct inaccuracies when possible. Keep people informed of why decisions have been made. The themes of procedural justice again take center stage as we strive to help others understand the logic behind the distribution of reward outcomes.

Equity theory also underscores the importance of leaders taking stock to be sure that their decisions are objective, factually based and unbiased. For example, it is not uncommon for leaders to develop closer associations with some colleagues than others — an observation that has spawned an entire tract of research known as leader-member exchange theory.[22]

Not surprisingly, the small "inner circle" receives a disproportionate amount of the leader's time and attention, especially when compared with others. Those outside the inner circle often feel that special privileges, plum assignments and confidential sharing occurs between the leader and those in the inner circle. And, unfortunately, research suggests that they are often correct in these assessments. This awareness should raise the bar of equity concerns. We encourage leaders to make special efforts to reach out, communicate and include those outside the inner circle to help thwart perceptions of inequity.

Goal Setting Theory

Goal setting theory offers several important themes.[23] This theory argues that clear, specific and challenging goals lead to higher performance than nonspecific "do your best" goals. The logic is straightforward. Without clarity and specificity, action is unfocused and efforts are fragmented. If goals lack challenge and are too easily attained, motivational potential is stagnated. Conversely, if goals are perceived as being too difficult to attain, individuals may not strive for them. With these precepts in mind, we recommend "stretch" goals — those that are experienced as realistic challenges.

Of course, goals only lead to higher performance when they are accepted by our people. Research has shown that goal acceptance can be enhanced in two primary ways: making goals public, and thereby increasing one's level of accountability,[24] and involving people in the goal setting process.[25] By doing so, individuals take ownership of their goals and feel like they have greater control over their work environment.

Although involvement is critical, individuals should not unilaterally set their own goals. There are two reasons for this caveat. First, as noted above, goals lead to high performance when the goals are challenging. Leader involvement helps assure the establishment of genuine stretch goals. Second, you need to make sure that others' goals are consistent with your vision, the organizational mission and other interlocking goals.[26]

Expectancy Theory

While research supports our discussion of motivation so far, there will be situations when your efforts do not result in higher employee performance. At times, we become aware that an individual's motivation has waned or slipped. Expectancy theory is a powerful diagnostic tool for these situations.[27]

According to expectancy theory, motivation is a function of three interacting cognitive interpretations. The first of these assessments is known as the "effort-to-performance" expectancy. Here, individuals must believe (a reasonable probability or likelihood) that if they put in effort, they will be able to reach designated performance goals. Logically, without such a belief, motivation is lost.

The second assessment is known as the "performance-to-outcome" expectancy. Here, individuals must believe that if they reach performance goals, desired and promised outcomes (rewards) will be forthcoming. Again, if one does not believe this, motivation is diminished.

Third, individuals must value the rewards that are being offered, which generally means that these rewards are salient or important within their current need structure. Even if people believe they can reach performance and that rewards will be delivered, motivation falls if the reward holds little or limited value for the individual at hand.

In most cases, a low performance-to-outcome expectancy arises from a lack of trust. This distrust may be targeted toward a leader who repeatedly has failed to deliver on promised rewards. Or, the distrust may be organizationally focused — a view that because of competitive factors, the organization will not deliver on promised reward outcomes. These expectancy perceptions are fragile. They may turn on rumors and misinformation. Yet diagnosing this issue and the expectancy breakdown provides the leader a path of remediation — generally to enhance communication and dispel the foundations of mistrust.

In a similar manner, if we determine that depleted motivation is because of the presence of low or undervalued rewards, a path of action may be set. Perhaps incentive systems have become stale, outdated and out of sync with the best practices in the industry. As noted earlier, the best way to know what our people value as a reward is by having interpersonal connections, knowing their values and understanding their personal and career aspirations.

We recently worked with a promising, young financial analyst within a hospital system. A hard charger, he was recognized for both his outstanding contributions and his impressive work effort. Over the last six months, something changed. Although his work remained solid, his drive, intensity and willingness to "go the extra mile" was somehow different.

Aware of his restlessness and rising discontent, his director made sure that he received the highest incremental salary adjustment that the system allowed. Of course, the young man gratefully accepted the increase, but there was no bump in his level of energy or motivation. Talking openly and candidly, the director was able to uncover a valued outcome, one that is increasingly prevalent among young, talented people. He wanted more "growth opportunities" — chances to learn and expand his formidable skills.

Wisely fearing she may lose this young man, the director offered him a role on a recently formed team to explore new acquisitions for the system. Here, the young man's talents were in full gear; he met and interacted with leaders throughout the hospital system and he grew. Once again, he was back to the work ethic that others had come to expect, and he loved what he was doing.

While performance-to-outcome assessments and outcome-value assessments are important, the effort-to-performance expectancy may provide the most striking challenges. Here, leaders begin to explore the possible breakdowns and pitfalls. A low effort-to-performance expectancy is generally because of a person's perception of lacking the capacity to perform or a lack of confidence.

Capacity usually revolves around resource issues. The individuals may not believe they have the skills, knowledge, understanding, background, available resources or time needed to be successful. Leaders must judge the veracity of such concerns. If skill deficiency is truly the issue, training and development may be in order.

More problematic, however, can be issues of confidence. Confidence or self-efficacy — one's belief in his or her ability to accomplish a given task — has been an important arena of behavioral research and insight.[28] For example, we understand that individuals who have a high self-efficacy tend to set high goals and persist in the face of setbacks, and thus have higher performance in the workplace than their counterparts with lower self-efficacy.[29]

So the question then becomes, how might a leader build a follower's self-efficacy? The most powerful way to build self-efficacy is through "mastery" or successive success. In theory, experiences of success increase efficacy. Of course, we may need to help our people recognize and appreciate their successes, and we may need to help them refrain from a debilitating tendency some have to trivialize or minimize their successes.

The second most effective way to increase self-efficacy is through vicarious experiences — being aware of others who are similar to us and who have been able to reach similar goals. As a result, people begin to reason, "I have the same talents and abilities as that other person who was able to accomplish this task, so I should be able to accomplish this task." Once this realization occurs, individuals start to believe in their own ability.

The third way to build self-efficacy is through verbal persuasion — the act of others encouraging and affirming that one is capable of task accomplishment. Here, it may be helpful for the leader to assure individuals by communicating genuine confidence in them.

Usually, leaders have to start with verbal persuasion and providing the follower with examples of vicarious experience. This will hopefully spark the process of building self-efficacy so that the follower will attempt to accomplish the given task. After the follower attempts to perform the task, and if they do not succeed, it is the leader's responsibility to point out what the follower did correctly, and what actions the follower needs to do to improve performance. The leader must celebrate the small success to build the efficacy through recognizing the mastery model.

Beyond Motivation — Inspiring Employees

Flow States

An intriguing area of research has emerged from Mihaly Csikszentmihalyi and his work on the motivating potential of "flow." Flow represents a state of total psychological emersion in a task.[30] While in these flow states, individuals are so focused on the task at hand that nothing else seems to matter. Flow states occur because individuals are performing tasks so challenging that they must use all of their psychological resources to accomplish the task. Stated differently, flow occurs when the demands and challenges of our work require the full use of our skills, talents and experiences, and these demands tap into our interests and passions.

Not surprisingly, flow states yield high levels of performance — remember, our skills and talents are being maximized. Further, flow states generate high levels of personal meaning and significance, presumably because our interests and passions are tapped and important accomplishments are occurring.

Here's the interesting thing about flow states. Individuals may not necessarily look forward to doing activities that put them into flow states, but once they hit a flow state and then exit that state, there is a strong internal drive to return to the flow state. For example, a surgeon may not look forward to performing a difficult surgery. She may even experience some level of anxiety about doing the surgery. However, once in the moment performing the surgery, she is completely focused. She does not think about the disagreement she had with her teenage son that morning or the hour-long commute home. She doesn't consider hospital politics or the never-ending scheduling conflicts. She is required in that moment to use all of her cognitive resources to perform a successful surgery. And when the surgery is over, she realizes a sense of inner peace that is the byproduct of being in a flow state. Even more important, she is looking forward to the next challenging surgery.

For an individual to obtain a flow state while performing a task, the task must have immediate feedback and it must challenge us to continue to improve. For instance, one of the reasons video games are "addictive" is that they have the basic elements that put people in flow states. There is immediate feedback in the form of points, and as soon as the player's ability matches the challenge of the game, the player moves to the next level with additional challenges.

As a leader, it is important to realize that as one's ability increases, the challenge of the work must also increase. Further, all work is multifaceted. Some parts of every job are rather mundane. However, opportunities to experience flow states, even for a limited segment of the day, can enhance motivation.

Job Shaping

In his bestselling book *Good to Great,* Harvard professor Jim Collins offers straightforward and foundational advice.[31] He argues that to build a winning organization, leaders must "get the right people on the bus" and "get them in the right seats." Without the right people — people who possess the skills and expertise to perform at high levels — hopes for performance are mere pipe dreams.

However, his second point is more nuanced. Given an array of talent, we must be able to get our people in the right roles — providing work opportunities that use their talents while contributing to organizational goals and mission. Traditionally, we slot people into our existing structure, presumably making "best-fit" decisions. However, in today's fast-changing climate, thinking more creatively may be helpful.

Marcus Buckingham has contributed a dynamic idea known as "job shaping."[32] Every job and every role has dimensions that are challenging and activating, as well as those that are necessary but mundane (patient notes do have to be done). Buckingham has argued for a different starting point. Let's look at the unique array of skills, talents and passions our people bring to the table. Let's consider rethinking and redesigning their work to give them the opportunity to do what they do best (and enjoy the most) more often.

Here, at least as much as we can, we are adjusting the job to the person rather than requiring the person to conform to the job. Pragmatically, there are always limits here, yet the consideration of job shaping can be powerful, especially when working with highly talented professionals.

Concluding Thoughts: The Case for Costless Motivation

Motivation does not need to focus on formal compensatory-based reward systems. Often, small and seemingly subtle exchanges can be powerful motivators. We recently sat with a brilliant young surgeon who was entering the arena of leadership. Discussing the topic of motivation, her focus was clear. "I will never forget the day that Dr. Jones (a respected senior surgeon) told me that I did very good work. And then, in his own goofy way, he showed me as much warmth as he could — a fist bump."

It all seems so simple — a brief statement and an awkward action. Yet it was remembered. This young surgeon felt a rush of personal significance that both affirmed her and drove her to excel.

There is amazing power in affirmation and sincere statements of praise and recognition. Many leaders, especially when working with highly trained professionals, provide too little affirmation, often out of a fear of providing too much. In attempting to discern why this occurs, two themes are apparent. First, many leaders are concerned that their attempts at affirmation will be seen as insincere, ingratiating or manipulative. Second, many of us have a fundamental belief that intelligent, field-specific experts clearly grasp the impact of their competence and contributions and neither need nor desire external validation.

Of course, lavish, unwarranted praise can have a boomerang effect, especially if insincerity is detected. So, we do too little. The need for affirmation remains and its motivating impact is untapped.

As discussed in an earlier chapter, affirmation and recognition have their greatest impact when three factors are applied. First, affirmations should be "earned" — some visible, clear and distinguishable action or outcome is the reason for the recognition. Second, the affirmation should be "timely"

— delivered soon enough that the reinforcement value of the affirmation is clearly associated with the desired behavior. Third, the affirmation should be "basic" — as opposed to over-the-top. In this manner, affirmation becomes part of your ongoing style. It can be as basic as "Thanks for all the extra work yesterday."

There is a further impact of judicious and sincere affirmations. They build perceptions of personal significance. Significance may be one of the most powerful motivators for any of us — that feeling that "I count; I am important and I make a difference." We gain our sense of significance from many sources, but none is more direct than earned affirmations.

In many ways, when we work to build relationships and foster stronger interpersonal connections — the essential foundations of this book — we build satisfying and motivating working environments and high-performing cultures. Work needs to be accomplished. High performance must be assured. These are absolutes and they cannot be mitigated. However, the building of powerful interpersonal relationships can and should coincide with and enhance our efforts to achieve top-flight performance. Edgar Schein, with both cynicism and realism, has noted, "We value task accomplishment over relationship-building and either are not aware of this cultural bias or, worse, don't care and don't want to be bothered by it."[33]

Each year *Fortune* magazine publishes its annual list of the "100 Best Companies to Work For." Researchers have culled these lists to determine what these companies do that others do not. How does one earn a designation as being the "best"? These organizations, through their leadership and throughout their ranks, created work environments that are rich in credibility, respect, fairness, pride and camaraderie.[34] Interestingly, these outcomes are the products of sensitivity of approach and the building of relationships as much as they are the delivery of the latest and greatest incentive plan.

....

1.   Lathan, G. P. (2012). *Work motivation: History, theory, research, and practice* (2nd ed.). Thousand Oaks: Sage. Locke, E.A. & Latham, G.P. (2004). What should we do about motivation theory? Six recommendations for the twenty-first century. *Academy of Management Review, 29*(3), 388-403. Steers, R.M., Mowday, R.T., Shapiro, D.L. (2004). The future of work motivation theory. *Academy of Management Review, 29*(3), 379-387.

2.   Anderson, N.H., & Butzin, C.A. (1974). Performance = motivation x ability: An integration-theoretical analysis. *Journal of Personality and Social Psychology, 30*(5), 598. Heider, F. (1958). *The Psychology of Interpersonal Relations*. New Jersey: Lawrence Erlbaum Associates.

3. LePine, J.A.; LePine, M.A., & Jackson, C.L. (2004). Challenge and hindrance stress: Relationships with exhaustion, motivation to learn and learning performance. *Journal of Applied Psychology, 98*, 883-891. Stoner, C.R., & Stoner, J.S. (2013). *Building Leaders: Paving the path for emerging leaders.* New York: Routledge.

4. Freud, S. (2012). *The Future of an Illusion.* Ontario, Canada: Broadview Press.

5. Maslow, A.H. (1943). A theory of human motivation. *Psychological Review, 50*(4), 370-396. Maslow, A.H. (1954). *Motivation and Personality.* New York: Harper and Row.

6. Alderfer, C.P. (1969). An empirical test of a new theory of human needs. *Organizational Behavior and Human Performance, 4*(2), 142-175. Barnes, L.B. (1960*). Organizational Systems and Engineering Groups.* Boston: Harvard Graduate School of Business. Harrison, R. (1966). *A Conceptual Framework for Laboratory Training.* Washington, DC: National Training Laboratory.

7. Barnes, L.B. (1960). Harrison, R. (1966).

8. Hackman, J.R,. & Oldman, G.R. (1976). Motivation through the design of work: Test of a theory. *Organizational Behavior and Human Performance, 16*(2), 250-279. Hackman, J.R., & Oldman, G.R. (1980), *Work redesign* (Vol. 72). Reading, MA: Addison-Wesley.

9. Human, L.J., & Biesanz, J.C. (2011). Through the looking glass clearly: Accuracy and assumed similarity in well-adjusted individuals' first impressions. *Journal of Personality and Social Psychology, 100*(2), 349-364.

10. Alvanzo, A.H., Cohen, G.M., & Nettleman, M. (2003). Changing physician behavior: Half-empty or half-full? *Clinical Governance, 8*(1), 69-78.

11. Henning-Schmidt, D., & Wiesen, D. (2014). Other-regarding behavior and motivation in health care provision: An experiment with medical and non-medical students. *Social Science and Medicine, 108*, 156-165.

12. Robinson, G.F.; Switzer, G.E.; Cohen, M.E.D.; Primack, B.A.; Kapoor, W.N.; Seltzer, M.D., … Rubio, D.M. (2013). A shortened version of the Clinical Research Appraisal Inventory: CRAI-12. Academic medicine: *Journal of the Association of American Medical Colleges, 88*(9), 1340-1345.

13. Trisolini, M. (2011). Introduction to pay for performance. In Trisolini, M.S.; Pope, G.C.; Mitchell, J.B., & Greenwald, L.M. *Pay for Performance in Health Care: methods and approaches* (Vol. 1, pp. 8-28). Triangle Park, NC: RTI Press.

14. Cassel, C.K., & Jain, S.H. (2012). Assessing individual physician performance: Does measurement suppress motivation? *Journal of the American Medical Association, 307*(24), 2595-2596.

15. Stajkovic, A.D., & Luthans, F. (1997). A meta-analysis of the effects of organizational behavior modification on task performance, 1997-1995. *Academy of Management Journal, 40*(5), 1122-1149.

16. Luthans, F., & Kreitner, R. (1985). *Organizational behavior modification and beyond: An operant and social learning approach.* Chicago, IL: Scott Foresman & Co.

17. Deci, E.L., & Ryan, R.M. (1985). Cognitive evaluation theory. *Intrinsic Motivation and Self-Determination in Human Behavior,* (pp. 43-85). New York: Springer Publishing Co.

18. Kiran, T., Wilton, A. S. Moineddin, R., Paszat, L., & Glazier, R. H. (2014). Effect of payment incentives on cancer screening in Ontario primary care. *The Annals of Family Medicine, 12*(4), 317-323.

19. Pink, D.H. (2011). *Drive: The surprising truth about what motivates us.* New York: Penguin.

20. Chaix-Coutrier, C., Durand-Zaleski, I., Jolly, D., & Durieux, P. (2000). Effects of financial incentives on medical practice: Results from a systematic review of the literature and methodological issues. *International Journal for Quality in Health Care, 12*(2), 133-142.

21. Adams, J.S. (1963). Toward an understanding of inequity. *Journal of Abnormal and Social Psychology,* 67, 422-436. Mowday, R.T. (1996). Equity theory predictions of behavior in organizations. In Steers, ;Porter, , & Bigley, (Eds.). *Motivation and Leadership at Work* (6th ed.). New York: McGraw-Hill.

22. Graen, G.B. & Uhl-Bien, M. (1995). The relationship-based approach to leadership: Development of LMX theory over 25 years. *Leadership Quarterly, 67*(2), 219-247.

23. Locke, E.A. & Latham, G.P. (2002). Building a practically useful theory of goal setting and task motivation: A 35-year odyssey. *American Psychologist, 57*(9), 705.

24. Locke, E.A., Shaw K.N., Saari, L.M. & Latham, G.P. (1981). Goal setting and task performance: 1969-1980. *Psychological Bulletin, 90*(1), 125-152.

25. Erez, M.; Earley, P.C., & Hulin, C.L. (1985). The impact of participation on goal acceptance and performance: A two-step model. *Academy of Management Journal, 28*(1), 50-66.

26. Schneider, B.; Brief, A.P., & Guzzo, R.A. (1996). Creating a climate and culture for sustainable organizational change. *Organizational Dynamics, 24*(4), 7-19.

27. Vroom, V.H. (1964). *Work and Motivation.* New York: Wiley. Lawler, E.E.; Suttle, J.L. (1973). Expectancy theory and job behavior. *Organizational Behavior and Human Performance, 9*(3), 482-503.

28. Bandura, A. (1977). Self-efficacy: Toward a unifying theory of behavioral change. *Psychological Review, 84*(2), 191.

29. Bandura, A. (1986). *Social Foundations of Thought and Action: A social cognitive theory.* Englewood Cliffs, NJ: Prentice-Hall. Stajkovic, A.D., & Luthans, F. (1998). Self-efficacy and work-related performance: A meta-analysis. *Psychological Bulletin, 124*(2), 240.

30. Csikszentmihalyi, M. (1990). *Flow: The psychology of optimal performance.* New York: Cambridge University Press.

31. Collins, J. (2001). *Good to Great: Why some companies make the leap ... and others don't.* New York: Harper Collins.

32. Buckingham, M. (2005). What great managers do. *Harvard Business Review, 83*(3), 70-79.

33. Shein, E. A, (2013). *Humble Inquiry: The gentle art of asking instead of telling.* San Francisco: Berrett-Koehler, p. 55.

34. Burchell, M. & Robin, J. (2011). *The Great Workplace: How to build it, how to keep it, and why it matters.* San Francisco: Jossey-Boss.

9

Change: A Future of Opportunity

....

MEDICAL PIONEER HANS SELYE IS GENERALLY ACKNOWLEDGED as the father of modern stress research. His foundational general adaptation syndrome; his differentiation of eustress and distress; and his logic of stress' curvilinear impact on performance are established foundations of the field. Queried as to how one could avoid stress, Selye retorted that, "No one can live without some degree of stress all the time."[1] His message was clear and direct — short of death, efforts to avoid stress were fruitless.

Selye's response provides an apt introduction to the topic of change. The inevitable dynamics of change affect every individual, team and organization. Indeed, adaptation and transition define human existence, personal growth and organizational survival. To paraphrase Selye, the only organizational system that is immune from the swirl of change is one that has already failed. And yet strangely and paradoxically, we are also reminded of the words of poet W.H. Auden, "We would rather be ruined than changed." Economist John Kenneth Galbraith offered his own bleak perspective, with a more interpersonal tone: "Faced with the choice between changing one's mind and proving there is no need to do so, almost everyone gets busy on the proof."[2]

In many ways, this entire book has been about change. Both the external environment of the health care industry and your immediate organizational context drive and demand change. Further, as we live with the formidable challenges facing health care, it is clear that the important changes we envision will be radical departures from the status quo, replete with new priorities and course-changing initiatives.[3] Because of the uncertainty, volatility and turbulence involved, these changes will be experienced as disruptive (as opposed to benign) in nature. In turn, it is reasonable to expect emotions of resistance from those involved.

As leaders, you envision change as a "solution" — an answer to some problem that must be rectified. As visionaries, you also see change as an "opportunity" — a bold movement of progress that furthers some noble cause that is congruent with enhancing your central mission. As pragmatists, you accept that you must confront, challenge and alter the status quo.[4] However, it will come as no surprise that leaders and employees often view change quite differently.[5] What appears as a logical and creative strategic necessity from the leader's point of view can be perceived as an unwarranted, unnecessary and poorly conceived disruption to those working deeper in the organizational structure.

The proverbial plot thickens. While we, as leaders, clearly grasp the need for change and readily extol the merits that will be gleaned from experiencing its fulfillment, a harsh reality looms. As we noted in an earlier chapter, research indicates that the majority of the change initiatives that are started each year fail, and up to 90 percent of these initiatives fall so far short of initial expectations that they simply cannot be viewed as complete successes.[6]

Part of this damning scenario is because of the all-too-familiar culprit of "initiative decay." Here, new initiatives are introduced in a burst of enthusiasm, laden with promise. Yet, as the days and months pass, the central tenets seem to be ignored and abandoned; organizational efforts and energies drift and the initiative "peters out," only to be replaced by the next iteration — a freshly minted, latest-and-greatest change initiative.[7]

Initiative decay has a pervasive effect, especially when it is experienced repeatedly. It fosters a mindset where people expect initiatives to lack stability and drift away. As such, new approaches and creative working methods fail to garner the commitment that is necessary to become ingrained within the normative structure of the organization.[8] In addition, having previously experienced initiative decay, organizational members are reluctant to embrace new changes that are seen as troubling and controversial. They reason — correctly — that if they resist long enough, the initiative will diminish and be abandoned. In this manner, a pattern of initiative failure and a lack of sustainability becomes embedded in the collective psyche.

There is a deeper motivational impact at play. Confronted with a barrage of ever-mounting calls for change, people begin to approach each impending initiative with a sense of ambivalence.[9] Motivation flounders and people "work to task," doing only what they must but injecting neither a sense of deep commitment nor psychological ownership.

In the face of this troubling and confusing scenario, we search for clarity and understanding. What is going on? How is it possible that our best leaders — our best minds — continually create and deploy a series of problematic change initiatives? How can the mark be missed so often?

There is little doubt that some initiatives fail because of poorly conceived strategies. Yet this is generally not the case. Most leaders are quite adept at assessing critical strategic drivers and crafting meaningful visions that are coupled with well-reasoned direction and thoughtful, impactful initiatives. Let's be clear, in most cases, the deficiencies that precede initiative decay and failure are not with the plan.

Instead, the devil is in the detail — the execution of the plan. Even the best of plans spins toward failure when the nuances and complexities of effective execution are given too little attention. And, as we will see, these complexities are almost always interpersonal in nature.

The case developed above may seem obvious. Yet, as patterns of shattered and inconsequential change initiatives attest, more is needed. Realistically, if change initiatives are to be viable and sustainable, leaders must assure that those involved in the process of change possess reasonable levels of commitment to the change, a theme that has received recent research attention.[10] Commitment to change involves at least three interlocking dynamics. Here, we must create a climate where those affected by change possess a positive attitude toward the change, possess a sincere "intention to support" the change and possess a willingness to work for the successful roll-out of the change.[11]

These three conditions require careful attention and point to a complex set of behavioral dynamics that are associated with the successful execution of change. Let's explore these dynamics in greater depth.

The Behavioral Dynamics of Change

Gaining commitment is best viewed from the micro, or personal, level. For those involved with change, it is always a personal issue. Cognitively and emotionally, each individual considers, "How will I be affected?" And there is an additional dynamic. We have long accepted that even among our most progressive organizations, strong pressures to maintain the status quo prevail.[12] This is both reasonable and logical, as the status quo represents an arena of understanding and comfort. Even when individuals do not like all elements of the current state, they have probably made adjustments and learned how to work most effectively within the current system.

In an insightful look at the difficulties with change, Chip and Dan Heath have depicted the two sides of change — a rational side and an emotional side.[13] They note what we all know through experience. As leaders, we are comfortable and skilled in building the analytically driven, rational "business case" for change. In fact, research suggests that careful consideration of the rational base has historically been the dominant, driving focus of organizational change efforts.[14] This certainly is the logical starting point — the critical necessity — as change must be grounded in a strong, pervasive and compelling rational foundation.

But there is also a practical, personal and emotional side to change. It is important to realize that organizational members may understand, at an intellectual level, the rational case for change. They may even grasp the indisputable competitive necessity that drives a new initiative. However, even such a change is experienced through a range of uncertain and troubling emotional themes.

The explanatory logic for emotional hesitancy is multifaceted. First, change — even needed and desired change — brings disruption at a time when many people perceive that "their plate is already full." One more adjustment, one more element of uncertainty and one more point of stress may seem too much to absorb. And deeper behavioral issues are often at stake. Anticipating change, people reason (and probably correctly so) that predictability will be diminished. Further, they surmise that their sense of control will be either threatened or dramatically disrupted. In many cases, recipients of change begin to question their sense of significance, trying to anticipate whether they will still be as valued and important in the new system as they are in the current one.

Two critical outcomes must be noted. First, careful consideration of both the rational and emotional sides of change is essential for commitment to change and initiative success.[15] Second, the emotional side of change can and frequently will overpower the rational side of change, leading to an unwillingness to support and work for change that eventuates as initiative decay and failure of promising change initiatives.[16] Shawn Achor has offered this succinct summary: "When challenges loom and we get overwhelmed, our rational brains get hijacked by emotions."[17]

Faced with the potential of emotional disruption and turmoil, many organizational members recoil into a series of behavioral responses that have broadly been characterized as "resistance to change." Resistance to change is often grossly misunderstood, and resisters are maligned and assigned unfortunate and unwarranted labels. We have all heard the attempts to browbeat resisters (and potential resisters) into submission by labeling them as aberrant. "He's stuck in the past." "She's a foot-dragger who just hates progress." "There is not a single forward-thinking bone in his body." Or one of our favorites, "She is too old and stuck in her ways to accept any change." In general, such labels are empirically inaccurate and behaviorally naive. For example, there is no credible evidence that one's age, position, experience or intelligence is logically related to a propensity to resist change.

We encourage you to consider an alternative view of resistance. Resistance is a normal human tendency, a psychologically healthy response to the perceived uncertainty and disruption that is taking place. It can be even be viewed expansively — as a signal that something is not quite right and needs more attention.[18] That something, quite often, ruminates in the emotional and behavioral realm. Research has long suggested that people resist out of fear — fear of losing something of value, fear of diminished status, fear of losing relationships, fear that I will lose some of my current power and influence, fear that I may not be as valued (significant) as I am now, and ultimately, fear that I might not be able to succeed.[19]

It is important for leaders to understand why and how resistance occurs. It is important to grasp the emotional underpinnings that form the base of resistance. And it is important to empathize with those affected by and experiencing feelings that manifest as resistance. These considerations are important because they help us respond and deal with the reality of resistance instead of pretending or hoping or assuming that resistance does not exist.

Indeed, most leaders can block or limit direct, overt expressions of resistance to change — essentially forcing people to suppress the emotional impact that they are feeling. Here, everyone smiles and nods at the leader, projecting a disguised tone of seeming approval and acceptance. Of course, suppressing resistance does not make it diminish or go away. It just becomes less visible, more likely to spark gossip and rumor and more likely to emerge with unexpected emotional gusto at a most inopportune time.

With these thoughts firmly in mind, we cannot and must not allow resistance to undermine and derail important and thoughtful change initiatives. As we often tell leaders in our workshops, we can understand resistance but we cannot be limited by it.

With an edge toward simplification, we know what generally happens as people are confronted with change. They pose, at least for internal rumination, three key questions: Why are we doing this? What exactly is going to happen? What will this mean for me? Leaders must help people navigate these questions. We will unpack these questions and the involved complexities in the remainder of this chapter in an effort to gain commitment and facilitate successful change.

Why: Building the "Compelling Case" for Change

Whether spoken or unspoken, most people approach change with a sense of cautious inquiry, searching for the underlying need — the "compelling case" — that is driving us from the status quo. Grasping the need and appreciating the logic will not guarantee acceptance and success. However, when people fail to understand the logic and fail to accept the compelling need for change, the likelihood of resistance and failure is greatly heightened.[20] Some scholars and thought leaders have boldly suggested that the compelling case is the most critical step in the process of change leadership.[21]

Harvard professor John Kotter has provided some of our most original and thoughtful work on change and the process of leading change. Kotter has popularized the significance of the compelling case by encouraging leaders to recognize, create and clearly demonstrate to others that a "sense of urgency" exists.[22] This sense of urgency is no benign phenomenon. Rather, it is the intense realization and conviction that if change does not happen, some deeply noxious negative outcome will eventuate. In short, unless there is change, "something bad will happen."[23]

Scholar and thought leader Edgar Schein addresses the compelling case with only slightly different verbiage, calling leaders to create a driving motivation for change by instilling a sense of "disequilibrium."[24] Schein's words are powerful. He notes that the presence of disequilibrium convinces people in the organization that goals are simply not being met and processes are not accomplishing what is desired and needed.

These themes, all ways of visualizing the compelling case, have even deeper impact. To build the compelling case, leaders must move — usually sequentially — through four stages.

First, as a leader, you must possess evidence that convinces you that change is absolutely necessary. We refer to this as the "unwavering conviction." Often, that evidence appears in the negative, as important outcome metrics show consistent, unacceptable results. At other times, you recognize that changing environmental forces demand change. Here, you must drive change and challenge the status quo from an anticipatory perspective because of what looms on the horizon.

The leader's unwavering conviction is a necessary but insufficient factor in successful change. And this is a point that is frequently missed. Insightful, visionary perspectives of what can be and must be are hallmarks of creative leadership. But this is never enough.

Second, leaders must translate and communicate the unwavering conviction in a way that resonates with others in the organization. In essence, this is the heart of change — building and communicating the "resonating case," or sense of urgency or disequilibrium. This stage is nuanced and behaviorally complicated. Importantly, this step is not about describing the change. In fact, that temptation should be resisted at this early junction. Instead, this step focuses on convincing people of the essential need for change. Turning again to Kotter, he argues that we can demonstrate the resonating case by helping our people realize one of three conditions: the presence of a current crisis, the rising likelihood of an impending crisis or the presence of a timely opportunity that simply cannot be missed.[25]

Third, leaders must realize that the "informational" case is not enough. Our people must experience an "attitudinal shift." With emphatic clarity, you must convince people that the status quo is untenable. You must convince them that the outcomes of inactivity simply cannot be risked. We must move people at a deep level to sense and appreciate that we must displace the status quo.

This step is problematic and frequently short-circuited by leaders. In many ways, that makes sense. After all, leaders have been studying the drivers and themes of change for months. It all makes sense and seems so obvious. Yet building and selling the resonating case helps others "get their arms around the situation," feel the urgency and experience the attitudinal shift. To repeat our earlier assertion, leadership scholars generally concur that without the resonating case and the attitudinal shift, change initiatives will be victims of decay and failure.

Enter our fourth point. Building and selling a resonating case takes time and requires incremental and continued communication. We emphasize this predominant need by labeling this stage "communication loading." In most cases, our tendency during these early stages of change is to under-communicate when the opposite is needed. Evidence should be shared. People must have opportunities to ask questions and receive credible responses. And people must have time to absorb what has been shared.

Realistically, we will never be able to sell the resonating case to everyone. Yet a critical mass of people (perhaps 75 percent of those affected) must accept the resonating case or change lacks the foundation needed for meaningful progress. Behaviorally, we are building the foundations that enable people to experience and feel the commitment, motivation and desire to work for and support all that follows.

Like you, we have seen too many examples of stalled or ineffective change because too little time and attention was spent on the compelling case. Let's look, however, at a leader who recognized and engaged the process with success.

We recently worked with Lynn Smith, a relatively young physician leader who was tapped to lead a struggling segment of her hospital's business. The evidence was staggering. Outcome metrics had been missed (and significantly so) for the past two years. The unit's reputation had sagged precipitously. Some of the most talented physicians and clinicians chose to voluntarily leave the unit. Several important, high-potential opportunities had been missed or given short shrift. As she reported to us, "The state of the union is bleak."

Interestingly, while those in the unit were aware of recent struggles, few really knew or understood just how bleak the situation had become. They knew the bits and pieces that directly affected them but lacked the intensity of the big picture. Not surprisingly, part of this blind ignorance was because of the previous leader's combination of limited communication and abrasive defensiveness when pressed or asked to explain various missteps. (It is interesting to note that this leader, without exception, rationalized the departure of his talent base by asserting that the unit was better off without the lost colleagues.)

To her credit, Smith took the time to assemble the troops, present as much evidence as she possibly could, present her assessment, encourage others' perspectives and listen. She met collectively when possible, in smaller groups when convenient, and in some politically and emotionally charged situations, she met individually. Importantly, she kept the focus on "what is," and she built the case. This took time. But it was weeks, not months. And, in the end, a critical mass was convinced of the compelling case and the need for change.

Let's conclude this section with a crucial point. By building and selling the compelling case and helping your people embrace the attitudinal shift, the likelihood of retrenchment and decay is reduced. Even when the dynamics of change execution become difficult (and they most certainly will), our people realize that going back is not an option. Even in the midst of disruption, they recall that the current state is unacceptable and competitively dangerous. And if they do not remember? We remind them.

What: Setting the Direction

Extensive literature exists regarding setting the direction of change.[26] We will not delve deeply into this theme other than to highlight three important and prevailing behavioral perspectives.

First, leaders must be visible "thought champions" of change. Jim Kouzes and Barry Posner have offered insight language, encouraging leaders to "envision the future," "become a futurist" and "inspire a shared vision."[27] Indeed. Leaders must offer challenging and credible possibilities. Remember that people are already primed to consider paradigm-busting moves because the compelling case has been firmly established and hopefully embraced.

Yet leaders should demonstrate strength of character and self-confidence by encouraging others to dissect and consider the credibility and veracity of the leader's possibilities. And this leads to our second perspective — the "involvement of others." Evidence clearly indicates the value and positive impact of involving others in the process of crafting the vision, as well as delineating supporting strategies and action plans.[28] Through involvement, we gain critical input and foster multiple sources of ownership. Involvement enhances familiarity, increases one's identification with the change and makes the change less daunting.[29] Involvement, inherently, is a statement of respect and trust. Involvement, inevitably, will reveal blind spots that must be considered and addressed. And involvement increases the likelihood that change will be accepted and implemented.

Unfortunately, too many leaders approach the direction and design of change as a "one-person show," apparently either believing that the best ideas are the exclusive purview of those in the seats of leadership; others in the organization have little interest in or desire to be part of shaping the change initiative; and/or involvement will lead to costly delays that stagnate needed action. Points one and two are fundamentally incorrect, and point three need not occur with proper team leadership and process management.

Moving unilaterally, without appropriate involvement, leaders also run the risk of "backsliding." Here, the leader charges ahead, driving pet initiatives, only to realize too late that others are lagging behind in staggering displays of ambivalence or resistance. Playing "catch-up" by seeking out more active involvement in the face of a stalled initiative may be the only reasonable option. However, the leader will have already experienced diminished credibility and labels of arrogance.

Third, leaders must assure a "coherence of attention." It is the leader's charge to encourage input. And it is the leader's responsibility to meld this input into a unified plan that people can understand and rally behind. This theme becomes critical in the arena of rapid change. It is likely that your organization has many moving parts with a series of change initiatives in various stages of development and emergence.

Under such conditions, it is easy for people to become confused and disaffected. We hear the telltale signals of frustration. "We have too many things going on at once." "They're (leaders) expecting us to undo everything at once." Or, consider the insightfully telling perception, "The right hand does not know what the left hand is doing." All of these statements point to the same conclusion. Despite the need or efficacy of the work that is being done, the swirl of change lacks coherence. Amid this change, we emphasize the comments of Daniel Goleman: "The primary task of leadership is to direct attention."[30] Leaders must offer focus. They must help people sense how the parts fit together. By providing attention and focus and coherence of action, leaders must fight the potentially debilitating perception that "everything is a chaotic blur."

Personal Impact: Understanding and Managing Disruptions

Many conceptions of the various types of organizational change are present in the literature, and each possess merit. Some have encouraged us to view change through the lens of the degree of adaptation or innovation that will be required.[31] Others use terms such as *broad* and *radical,* differentiating these from their smaller, more easily accepted counterparts.[32]

As presented in Table 9-1, we offer a slight variation that is predicated on the emotional dynamics presented earlier in this chapter. Drawing from both theoretical and empirical strands, we view change according to its perceived disruption from the status quo.[33] To a large extent, our perspectives are applications and adaptations of the transactional theory of stress.[34] Let's delineate this logic carefully and, in the process, provide some leadership action points.

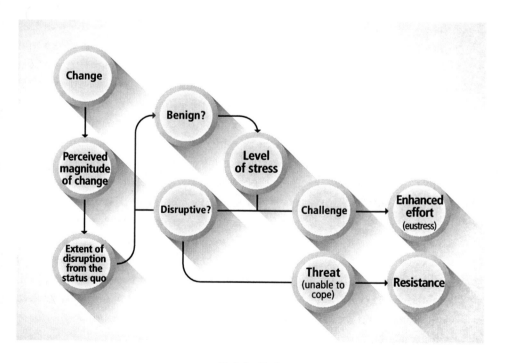

Table.9.1

Encountering change, people gauge its magnitude by assessing the "extent of disruption from the status quo" that will be created by the initiative at hand.

Of course, like so many of the interpersonal themes we have discussed, this assessment is a perception laden with all the biases that accompany any perceptual process. Unfamiliarity breeds perceptions of wide disruption. Lack of communication almost always leads to assumptions of sweeping disruptions. At this point, let's just note the obvious. Careful, early and ongoing communications can help us manage perceptions and avoid unnecessary concerns.

In most cases, when communication is limited, people move toward the worst-case scenario and assume the change will be more disruptive than it actually is. Consider a rather basic example that would be laughable if it were not so sad.

A few years ago, we were asked to talk with the security team of a regional hospital. The hospital's administration was in the final stages of establishing a contract with an outside agency to provide some basic services that had previously been required of the security department. Assuming that those in security would be delighted to have some of their more mundane duties reassigned, the administration was shocked at the rumor-laden backlash that seemed to be occurring. As we met with representatives from security, the first question went straight to the point: "OK, how many of us are getting fired?"

There were no planned terminations, and the administration truly seemed to be undertaking the contract to allow security time for more vital activities. Yet nearly nothing had been conveyed to the employees. And, in the absence of credible data, perceptions of massive disruption flourished.

Realistically, however, in our current health care environment many of the planned and needed changes will be disruptive. But even disruptive change can be accepted with commitment and energy. As our model suggests, much of this has to do with the way people interpret the personal impact of the disruption. If the change initiative is perceived as a "challenge," it is likely that the change will be approached with intensity and "enhanced effort." Here, we draw from an impressive line of research, indicating that some degree of stress (eustress) can positively affect motivation and performance.[35]

Of course, the obverse to the "challenge" perception occurs as the situation turns problematic. When people encounter the disruption and believe that they will be unable to cope and adjust, they experience a "threat" rather than a "challenge." Rather than eustress, distress is likely.[36] And, as we have carefully defined earlier, the logical response to such a condition is resistance.

The leadership focus is obvious. How can we help our people encounter change while maximizing their sense of "challenge" and minimizing their sense of "threat?" Let's consider three key factors.

Ongoing Communication

Both evidence and best practices underscore the need for engaged, ongoing communication during change.[37] Frequent communication is the best vehicle for minimizing disruptive misinformation and rumors. It is a key factor in helping people feel connected during a time of uncertainty. It helps people reshape their sense of what change will mean — their new sense of meaning — in successive stages. It encourages perceptions of justice by appealing to the explanatory dynamics of procedural justice.

Often, leaders are reluctant to communicate until all the details of change have been worked out and all the answers have been delineated. The ensuing gap in communication can be destructive. People need frequent check-ins, even those that are simply brief progress updates. There is wisdom and reality in an oft-repeated commentary: What people don't know, they make up.

We know that during change, most people are trying to understand and make sense of their new and evolving organizational context.[38] Scholars have even noted that these "meaning voids" may be the most problematic aspect of change for the affected recipients.[39] In fact, major shifts and confusion about meaning will generally result in resistance.[40] And, there is a rich line of literature that speaks to the leader's need to provide "sense-giving" — carefully communicating new values, beliefs and expectations to help clarify what may be confused interpretations about what change will bring.[41]

There is a final factor that should not be diminished. It has to do with the transitional nature of many changes, and the need for "values clarity." Recall from Chapter 2 the groundbreaking work of William Bridges.[42] He asserted that change involves doing things differently, while transition involves the emotional and relational adjustment that is much more problematic. Importantly, Bridges helped us understand that transitions are composed of three stages: an ending; a neutral period, often laden with stress and uncertainty, and a new beginning. The ending is critical and it is often given too little attention. It involves all that is left behind and the psychological impact that such movement carries.

Understanding these behavioral factors points to the significance of "value clarity." Here, the leader helps to ensure the legitimacy of the change by emphasizing over and over again the fundamental values — the noble cause —being enhanced through the change. Here, leaders can also articulate the values that will not change, again providing direction and assurance. Indeed, this is part of sense-giving. But it also provides important assurance of what is expected and what will be rewarded.

Consider the following example that underscores the impact of open and ongoing communication. McKinsey & Co. reported a study of two hospitals, each of which created independent purchasing groups to reduce costs.[43] "At one hospital, the CEO and chief purchasing officer communicated bold expectations for the initiative, and stakeholders (that is, physicians) at every level were involved throughout it." However, at the second hospital, such communication and involvement was nonexistent. Leaders throughout the hospital were virtually silent about the change and its effects. The first hospital exceeded outcome expectations in less than a year, while the second hospital secured only half of the anticipated savings.

Giving Voice to Resistance

Earlier, we noted the value of listening to resistance, and again we under-score how important these activities can be in the overall process of ongoing communication. During change, leaders are well served by having meetings whose sole purpose is hearing what is on the minds of their people.

In all likelihood, there will be some uncomfortable carping that takes place. Yet the willingness to listen to resistance achieves at least three important outcomes. First, it provides an emotional outlet and a means of catharsis for people. They understand, in many cases, that their pent-up concerns are widely recognized and have been broadly considered. Remember, as stated earlier, we can be open to allowing some degree of release because the compelling case keeps us moving ahead. We love the phrasing offered by Jeanie Duck, suggesting that it is just fine to allow people to visit "pity city," as long as we make it clear that they cannot move in![44]

In addition, providing for open expressions of resistance offers several positive possibilities.[45] First, we have the capacity to increase the accuracy of the information that is being processed. The value here should never be under-played. In the bestselling change book *Switch*, the authors succinctly note that "what looks like resistance is often a lack of clarity."[46] Second, we often will learn about key problem areas that were unknown to us. Accordingly, we can address these issues before they thwart the progress of our change initiative. Third, by listening, we project empathy and concern to our people.[47] By providing authentic voice, people are more likely to accept and support the change.[48]

Capacity Enhancement

In some cases, the perception of threat arises from a legitimate fear that one will be unable to master the new skills and behaviors that change will require. This fear dynamic has been described as "learning anxiety" — "the feeling that I cannot learn the new behaviors or adopt new attitudes without losing a feeling of self-esteem or group membership."[49]

Leaders must address the reality of learning anxiety, and generally do so by emphasizing three factors. First, mechanisms must be put in place to provide the training and development that is needed to close gaps in skills and in overall understanding. Second, the avenues for accessing these developmental programs must be clear and not cumbersome. Third, and perhaps most critical, the social stigma associated with participating in this training and development must be minimized.

In a technology-dominated world, we readily understand that any innovation will be ineffective unless those for whom it is intended have the capacity and willingness to avail themselves of these opportunities. Viral connectivity enhances our reach and opportunity for impact but only if those involved possess the skills and disposition to assure effectiveness. Or consider the case for medical simulation — a dynamic technology-based educational method that enhances clinician exposure to a broad variety of medical situations while minimizing real-world risks. Even the most impressive simulation facilities achieve impact only when medical faculty have been given time and training to devote to the demands and challenges of simulation-based education.[50]

Accessibility

People need more points of connection during change, not fewer. People need more of your time during change, not less. People need greater access to you during change, not roadblocks and limitations. This is the time to increase your visibility, not decrease it. This is the time to walk the floors, not remain hunkered in your office. As leaders, juggling the evolving maze of complexity that accompanies change execution, each of these needs works against your perspectives, your inclinations and your agenda.

Yet we should never underestimate how fragile and tenuous people can become when confronted with major change. Out of fear of making a mistake or misstep, people may actually become overly cautious. And we should never underestimate the benefits of having access to you and other key leaders.

We worked with the physician leader of a specialty clinic as he traversed the fallout of a major reorganization that altered the long-standing departmental structure of the clinic, changed several reporting relationships and resulted in the dismissal of a handful of low-performing employees. As he walked from the clinic entrance to his office, the tension was palpable. Friendly smiles were replaced by quick, perfunctory nods of the head. The break room, normally populated by a few employees engaged in a good-natured exchange, was vacant. Staff answered questions, but without the casual warmth that was normally expressed.

Encouraging the leader to become more accessible, he countered that his people "just needed some time to come to grips with what had happened." While his comment was no doubt true, the "time" he alluded to does not need to occur without leader presence.

We reminded him of the sense of fear that often permeates organizations after such changes — a focused area of study known as survivor anxiety.[51] With some minimal prompting, he made it his practice to take at least two (and in some cases three) passes through the clinic each day — early morning as the day starts, midday and toward the end of the normal workday. We encouraged him to stop by the lunchroom about noon, where many employees congregated. There was no need to say much, just grab a cup of coffee and let them see you. Did all of this change everything? Did it completely refocus the experience of change? Certainly not. But it did make a difference.

Reinforce Early Successes

Kotter encourages leaders to celebrate wins, especially early, quick wins.[52] In this manner, you help assure people that the change in place makes sense and that it works. Further, such early celebrations reinforce the behaviors that have provided success and increase the chances that they will be further employed.

These early celebrations need not be over-the-top. In fact, they should not be. Two things are important. First, people must know with unmistakable clarity the behaviors and outcomes that are being celebrated. Second, people must understand that the pattern of success can be and should be continued.

Concluding Thoughts: A Mindset of Change

There is a final theme that is especially pertinent for the turbulent climate that you face. In many ways, this theme touches on our fundamental assumptions about the way change interacts with our organizational world. Here, scholars have argued for a shift in mindset — a shift that conceptualizes change as ongoing rather than episodic.[53] As such, we must understand and help our people realize that change is never over. Rather, change is continual, an ever-present demand of competitiveness and survival.

As an ongoing experience, we must help our people become comfortable with a new approach where strategies and organizational actions are more "informed approximations" that home in on moving targets rather than "linear paths" focused on a fixed end. A simple story may be helpful.[54]

A few years ago, on a beautiful backwoods hike with my wife, the problem unfurled. Deep into our adventure, she suddenly stopped, turned toward me and boldly asserted, "We're lost."

I tersely retorted that we were indeed "not lost."

"Well, do you know where we are?"

I admitted that I did not know exactly, but countered that was far different from being truly lost because I did have my trusty compass. "This is a very good compass, and I am a very good compass reader." Reading and plotting, I confidently turned her gaze toward a tall clump of trees in the far distance and said, "We move toward those trees, and we will get back to camp."

When she asked if I was sure, I said, "This is a very good compass, and I am a very good compass reader."

Our first obstacle came less than a quarter of a mile on our trek toward the trees. We encountered a steep cliff. As my wife smugly complained that I never said anything about a cliff, I simply admitted, "I did not know about the cliff, but I know where we need to head to reach camp."

Sliding down the cliff, we focused on the bank of tress along the horizon. Another quarter of a mile or so, we encountered water. I saw a small creek, but my wife saw a swirling and treacherous stream. Crossing it, I again admitted that this was unexpected but were progressing toward the trees. We moved ahead and, as predicted, safely reached our camp.

Two weeks later, on a consulting trip to Scottsdale, Arizona, I went for a brisk predawn run with a colleague. Winding our way through the town and enjoying a spirited conversation, we paused for a break. The darkness, the conversation, the unknown territory all played a part, but the outcome was clear. I had lost my bearings and had no idea how to get back to the hotel.

My running buddy was quick to the rescue. His running watch was really a GPS that provided an easy-to-follow and detailed guide for us to follow. Every turn was noted and every landmark was clear.

I have used these stories and their analogy-laden impact frequently during our workshops. It speaks to our mindset. When people are going through change, they want and dearly need the GPS. Yet the simple truth is this: All we really have, even the best among us, is the compass. Hopefully, it is a "very good compass," held by a "very good compass reader."

Leaders have a vision and a direction. But we do not know, and in today's world cannot be expected to know, every detail and every obstacle and every frustrating diversion that will arise along the way.

We must project the mindset of resiliency, assuring our people of confidence in our direction and in our ability to navigate the obstacles together in the name of our noble cause. And we must convey that we will trudge through the obstacles successfully, and together.

1. Selye, H. (1984). *The stress of life*. P. xv.

2. Auden, W.H. (1947). *The Age of Anxiety*. New York: Random House, p. 123. Galbraith, J.K. (1971). Economics, peace, and laughter. New York: Signet, p. 50.

3. Gioia, D.A.; Thomas, J.B.; Clark, S.M.; & Chittipeddi, K. (1994). Symbolism and strategic change in academia: The dynamics of sensemaking and influence. *Organization Science, 5*, 363-383.

4. Kouzes, J.M. & Posner, B.Z. (2002). *The Leadership Challenge*. San Francisco: Jossey-Bass.

5. Strebel, P. (1996). Why do employees resist change? *Harvard Business Review,* May–June, 86–92.

6. Beer, M., & Nohria, N. (2000). Cracking the code of change. *Harvard Business Review, 78*(3), 133-141. IBM Business Consulting Services. (2004). *Your turn: The global CEO study 2004.* Retrieved from http://www-05.ibm.com/no/news/publications/IBI. Karp, T., & Gelgo, T.I.T. (2009). Reality revisited: Leading people in chaotic change. *Journal of Management Development, 28*(2), 81-93.

7. Doyle, M.; Claydon, T.; & Buchanan, D. (2000). Mixed results, lousy processes: Contrasts and contradictions in the management experience of change. *British Journal of Management, 11*, 59-80.

8. Buchanan, D.; Fitzgerald, L.; Ketley, D.; Gollop, P.; Jones, J.L.; Lamont, S.S.; Neath, A.; & Whitby, E. (2005). No going back: A review of the literature on sustaining organizational change. *International Journal of Management Reviews, 7*(3), 189-205.

9. Piderit, S. K. (2000). Rethinking resistance and recognizing ambivalence: A multidimensional view of attitudes toward an organizational change. *Academy of Management Journal, 25 (4), 783–794.*

10. Fedor, D.B.; Caldwell, S.; & Herold, D.M. (2006). The effects of organizational changes on employee commitment: A multi-level investigation. *Personnel Psychology, 59*, 1-29. Hersovitch, L. & Meyer, J.P. (2002). Commitment to organizational change: Extension of a three-component model. *Journal of Applied Psychology, 87*, 474-487.

11. Herold, D.M.; Fedor, D.B.; Caldwell, S.; & Liu, Y. (2008). The effects of transformational and change leadership on employees' commitment to change: A multi-level study. *Journal of Applied Psychology, 93*(2), 346-357.

12. Kanter, R.M. (1983). *The Change Masters: Innovation and entrepreneurship in the American corporation.* New York: Simon & Schuster.

13. Heath, C. & Heath, D. (2010). *Switch: How to change when change is hard.* New York: Broadway Books.

14. Burke, W.W.; Lake, D.G.; & Paine, J.W. (Eds.). (2009). *Organizational change: A comprehensive reader.* San Francisco: Jossey-Bass.

15. Van de Ven, A.H. & Sun, K. (2011). Breakdowns in implementing models of organizational change. *Academy of Management Perspectives, 25*(3), 58-74.

16. Heath & Heath, 2010. Kotter, J.P. & Cohen, D.S. (2002). *The heart of change: Real-life stories of how people change their organizations.* Boston: Harvard Business School Publishing. Labianca, G.; Gray, B.; & Brass, D.J. (2000). A grounded model of organizational schema change during empowerment. *Organization Science, 11*, 235-257.

17. Achor, S. (2010). *The Happiness Advantage.* New York: Crown Business, p. 17.

18. Jick, T.D. (1993). *Implementing Change.* Burr Ridge, IL: Irwin.

19. Connor, D.R. (1995). *Managing at the Speed of Change: How resilient managers succeed and prosper where others fail.* New York: Villard Books.

20. Hiatt, J.M. (2006). *ADKAR: How to implement successful change in our personal lives and professional careers.* Loveland, CO: Prosci. Kotter, J. & Schlesinger, L. (1979). Choosing strategies for change. *Harvard Business Review, 57*, 106-114.

21. Hiatt, 2006. Kotter, J. (1996). *Leading Change.* Boston: Harvard Business School Press.

22. Kotter, 1996. Kotter, J.P. (200*). *A Sense of Urgency.* Boston: Harvard Business Press.

23. Schein, E.H. (2010). *Organizational culture and leadership* (4th ed.). San Francisco: Jossey-Bass, p. 301.

24. Ibid.

25. Kotter, J. (1995). Leading change: Why transformational efforts fail. *Harvard Business Review, 73*(1), 59-67.

26. For example, see Kornacki, M.J. & Silversin, J. (2012). *Leading Physicians Through Change: How to achieve and sustain results.* (2nd ed.). Tampa, FL: American College of Physician Executives.

27. Kouzes, J.M. & Posner, B.Z. (2002). The leadership challenge. (3rd ed.). San Francisco: Jossey-Bass.

28. Lawler, E.E. & Hackman, J.R. (1969). The impact of employee participation in the development of pay incentive plans: A field experiment. *Journal of Applied Psychology, 53,* 467-471. Sashkin, M. (1976). Changing toward participative management approaches: A model and methods. *Academy of Management Review, 1,* 75-86.

29. Manz, C.; Bastien, D.; & Hostager, T. (1991). Effective leadership during change: A bi-cycle model. *Human Resource Planning, 14*(4), 275-287.

30. Goleman, D. (2013). The focused leader: How effective executives direct their own — and their organizations' — attention. *Harvard Business Review, 91*(12), 50-60, p. 52.

31. Nutt, P.C. (1986). Tactics of implementation. *Academy of Management Journal,* June, 230-261.

32. Gioia, *et. al.,* 1994.

33. Fedor, D.B.; Caldwell, S. & Herold, D.M. (2006). The effects of organizational change on employment: A multi-level investigation. *Personnel Psychology, 59,* 1-29.

34. Lazarus, R.S. & Folkman, S. (1987). Transactional theory and research on emotions and coping. *European Journal of Personality, 1,* 141-169.

35. Leung, K.; Huang, K.; Su, C.; & Lu, L. (2011). Curvilinear relationship between role stress and innovative performance: Moderating effects of perceived support for innovation. *Journal of Occupational and Organizational Psychology, 84*(4), 741-758. Yerkes, R.M. & Dodson, J.D. (1908). The relationship of strength of stimulus to rapidity of habit-formation. *Journal of Neurology and Psychology, 18,* 459-482.

36. Barling, J.; Kelloway, E.K.; & Frone, M.R. (2005). *Handbook of Work Stress.* Thousand Oaks, CA: Sage. Selye', H. (1978). *The Stress of Life* (2nd ed.), New York: McGraw-Hill.

37. Allen, J.; Jimmieson, N.L.; Bordia, P.; & Irmer, B.E. (2007). Uncertainty during organization change: Managing perceptions through communication. *Journal of Change Management, 7,* 187-210. Fiss, P.C. & Zaja, E.J. (2006). The symbolic management of strategic change: Sensegiving via framing and decoupling. *Academy of Management Journal, 49,* 1173-1193. Salem, P. (2008). The seven communications reasons organizations do not change. *Corporate Communications: An International Journal, 13,* 333-348.

38. Weick, K.E. (1995). *Sensemaking in Organizations.* Thousand Oaks, CA: Sage.

39. Schein, E.H. (1996). Culture: The missing concept on organizational studies. *Administrative Science Quarterly, 41,* 229-240.

40. Labianca, G.; Gray, B.; & Brass, D.J. (2000). A grounded model of organizational schema change during empowerment. *Organization Science, 11,* 235-257.

41. Gioia, D.A.; Thomas, J.B.; Clark, S.M.; & Chittipeddi, K. (1994). Symbolism and strategic change in academia: The dynamics of sensemaking and influence. *Organization Science, 5,* 363-383. Smith, A.D.; Plowman, D.A.; & Duchon, D. (2010). Everyday sensegiving: A closer look at successful plant managers. *Journal of Applied Behavioral Science, 46*(2), 220-244. Vuori, T. & Vitaharju, J. (2012). On the role of emotional arousal in sensegiving. *Journal of Organizational Change Management, 25*(1), 48-66.

42. Bridges, W. (1991). *Managing Transitions: Making the most out of change.* Cambridge, MA: DaCapo Press.

43. LaClair, J.A. & Rao, R.P. (2002). Helping employees embrace change. *Insights and Publications.* McKinsey & Co. www.mckinsey.com/insights/organization/helping_employees_embrace_change, accessed February 15, 2015.

44. Duck, J. (1998). Managing change: The art of balancing. Harvard Business Review on Change (pp. 55–81). Boston: Harvard Business School Press.

45. Ford, J.D. & Ford, L.W. (2009). Decoding resistance to change. *Harvard Business Review, 87*(2), 99-104. Ford, J.D.; Ford, L.W.; & D'Amelio, A. (2008). Resistance to change: The rest of the story. *Academy of Management Journal, 33,* 362-377.

46. Heath & Heath, 2010. p. 15.

47. Bies, R.J. & Moag, J.S. (1986). Interactional justice: Communication criteria of fairness. In R.J. Lewicki; B.H. Sheppard; & M.H. Bazerman (Eds.). *Research on Negotiation in Organizations* (pp. 43-55). Greenwich, CT: JAI Press. Tyler, T.R. & Bies, R.J. (1990). Interpersonal aspects of procedural justice. In Carroll, J.S. (Ed.). *Applied Social Psychology and Organizational Settings* (pp. 77-98). Hillsdale, NJ: Erlbaum.

48. Greenberg, J. (1994). Using socially fair treatment to promote acceptance of a worksite smoking ban. *Journal of Applied Psychology, 79,* 288-297.

49. Schein, 2010, p. 302.

50. Okuda, Y.; Bryson, E.O.; DeMaria Jr., S.; Jacobson, L.; Quinones, J. Shen, B.; & Levine, A.I. (2009). The utility of simulation in medical education: What is the evidence. *Mount Sinai Journal of Medicine, 76,* 330-343.

51. Noer, D.M. (2009). *Healing the Wounds: Overcoming the trauma of layoffs and revitalizing downsized organizations.* San Francisco: Jossey-Bass.

52. Kotter, 1996.

53. Weick, K.E. & Quinn, R.E. (1999). Organizational change and development. *Annual Review of Psychology,* 50, 361–386.

54. We presented a version of this example in an earlier book. Stoner, C.R. & Stoner, J.S. (2013). *Building Leaders: Paving the path for emerging leaders.* New York: Routledge.

10

Tomorrow: A Case for Possibility

....

T HROUGHOUT THESE CHAPTERS, WE HAVE OFFERED A PANORAMA
of some of the challenges confronting physician leaders — demands that
are intensified by the turbulence of today's health care context. You know
these dynamics well, as you live them every day. You face new and confusing
realities — opportunities, possibilities and dangers that are clouded with uncertainty. We have built the case that it is precisely because of the conflicting and
paradoxical nature of what lies ahead that leadership —enlightened, engaged,
difference-making physician leadership — is so deeply needed.

Within our shifting environment, the need for resiliency becomes paramount. We experience it at the macro-level. For example, Gary Hamel and Liisa
Valikangas have noted that organizational resilience — where organizations
read their environments and realign their resources more quickly than their
competitive rivals — is today's ultimate competitive advantage.[1]

The need for organizational resilience among our health care institutions
has never been more pressing nor more blatantly absent. As one physician
shared, "I have ideas. I think I know things that could be done — how policies and approaches could be improved. And I have absolutely no confidence
that any of it will ever happen within the hierarchy and procedurally laden
environment of my hospital."

At the micro-level — where all battles are fought and won (or lost) — resiliency is personal. As we addressed in the preceding chapter, it deals with
status-quo shattering disruption, perceived threats, adversity and a seemingly
constant calls to adapt and change. We have even suggested that the mindset
of ongoing change is the new reality — the new normal.

At times, the stories we hear are dramatic. We recall meeting with Don Mitchell, a 50-year-old physician who was part of a successful practice. Dejected and seemingly beaten down, Mitchell kept repeating one word — a word that described his interactive tone and his emotional state — *disillusioned*. He was disillusioned with his partners, who he felt were chasing the wrong goals, and with patient care receiving an ever-lowered sense of priority. He was disillusioned with the entire practice and its future, as it sat at the precipice of acquisition by a large hospital system. He spoke of disillusionment with his career — caught in the throes of too much red tape that drained meaning and significance from his work. And, not surprisingly, he was disillusioned with leaders who seemed to move to the latest and loudest edict rather than carve a path of clarity and purpose.

Unfortunately, we know that Mitchell is not unique. Research has indicated that a striking percentage of physicians are so discouraged with the current state of health care that they have considered leaving medical practice altogether.[2] And, as noted by Mary Jane Kornacki and Jack Silversin, "Among physicians, disenchantment with their chosen profession continues to grow."[3]

During these times of rapid change, what must leaders do? How can we help our people become part of the transformation, part of the journey, part of the quest for new possibilities? We carefully craft and enact the best practices of change management. And yet, the questions persist.

We sense that people are not really looking for a single, definitive answer. Indeed, there is none. Rather, they want a foundation or grounding from which further reflective thought may build. So we shift just a bit and turn toward three philosophical themes.

First, during times of chaotic volatility, people dearly need leaders who provide hope. Hope is a quality of resilience. It is not a blind, head-in-the-sand rendition that all is fine. Hope asks for neither naïveté nor the cheerleading of hype. Hope is centered and it is realistic. Hope demands an honest appraisal of reality. And it requires a vision of possibility. The structures and considerations of the preceding chapter were efforts to offer direction, clarity, decisiveness, communication and hope.

There is a second theme. Leaders, through their actions and demeanor, must "focus their attention toward others." Accordingly, leaders must pursue a purpose, or a cause, or a set of noble outcomes that extend beyond themselves. Scott Peck has noted that, for mentally healthy people, the needs of others are more important than their own gratification.[4]

That is quite a statement and it is a sophisticated and advanced form of leadership. In essence, this perspective indicates that the growth and development of others is the dominant need that one should pursue. In fact, this drive — this need — must supersede self-interest and self-domination. Such thinking is profound; it is foundational and it is a center pole of helping others navigate troubling movements of change.

But there is a third theme, powerful and perhaps controversial. Leaders must display compassion. Many people blanch at the warm and fuzzy emotions that emanate from a serious discussion of leader compassion. They eschew the compassionate leader by drawing a false dichotomy — suggesting an improbable coexistence between compassionate concern and regard for others and the drive for competitive performance and overall effectiveness. Yet compassion need not reduce leader objectivity. Leaders can display both compassion and decisiveness, and our best leaders have the capacity for both.

For many, the seeds of compassion seem inherent. For example, management philosopher Charles Handy has said, "We were not meant to stand alone. We need to belong — to something or someone. Only where there is a mutual commitment will you find people prepared to deny themselves for the good of others."[5] Important recent scholarship concurs with Handy, suggesting that rather than being predominantly self-serving, most of us are inherently kind, compassionate, empathic, cooperative and other-serving.[6]

Many perspectives and definitional themes surface when we consider compassion. In powerful words, Karen Armstrong has asserted that compassion "dethrones the ego from the center of our lives and puts others there."[7] There is a further notion — compassion "honor(s) the inviolable sanctity of every single human being, treating everybody, without exception, with absolute justice, equity and respect."[8] Herein lies our focus. Compassion is a facet of authenticity — the capacity to demonstrate genuine interest in and sensitivity to the needs of our people.[9] Researchers at the Center for Creative Leadership have included "compassion and sensitivity" among their key leadership competencies for executive success.[10]

Organizational scholars have explored the role of compassion in organizations, both from micro (individualistic) and macro (organizational) perspectives.

Here, researchers have viewed compassion as a dynamic process, composed of three sub-processes: "noticing" — becoming aware of another's pain;

"feeling" — experiencing an emotional reaction to that pain, and "respond-ing" — engaging in action.[11] Critically, these authors suggest that compassion moves from the individual to organizational level when the sub-processes are "legitimized within an organizational context and propagated among organizational members ... (and) coordinated across individuals."[12]

Pragmatically, our discussion of compassion must consider two types of compassion as "emotional compassion" and "engaged compassion." Emotional compassion is what we feel in the face of another's plight. As such, emotional compassion requires that we experience both a personal awareness of an-other's condition and that we have feelings for what they are experiencing. Some argue that the feeling we have is one of pity or distress. We prefer to think more expansively and describe this feeling, in its desired form, as "genuine concern."

Leaders can (and some do) take steps to seclude and inoculate themselves from awareness. Consequently, when stabbed with striking evidence of real concerns within their units and organizations, they seek absolution with the "I had no idea" refrain.

While leaders may rarely have a truly unvarnished view of what their people are experiencing, compassionate leaders seek to break down the barriers of distance through openness, transparency, connection, visibility and accessibility. They also have an amazing capacity to accept feedback receptively and non-defensively.

Engaged compassion moves from awareness and concern to action. Action is different. While we may concede that awareness and empathy generally precede action, the former two conditions do not necessarily lead to the third.

We would be naïve to ignore the risks that are involved when moving from emotional to engaged compassion. Foremost, we are almost always unsure of how others will respond, regardless of the depth of our concern or the quality of our intentions. Here, logic prevails. The better we know someone, the more interactions that have taken place, the greater empathy that has been built, the greater the interpersonal trust, and the more open we have been with expressions of feelings in the past, the greater the likelihood that acts of compassion will be perceived as helpful and positive. In short, engaged compassion has a better chance of being beneficial when positive interpersonal dynamics have been ingrained and are part of the relational dynamics between parties.

Concluding Thoughts: The Art and the Journey

As we conclude this book, we want to highlight two points for consideration as you continue down the path of leadership. First, we remind you that leadership is an art. There are things that *do* work and things that *don't* work in the practice of leadership; and our hope is that this book has provided you with some of those ins and outs.

In this book, we have focused on empirical and theoretical research to guide our views on how leaders should navigate the complexities of interpersonal dynamics, but you, of course, are your own person. You have your own unique personality and characteristics. Leadership does not come with a "one size fits all" solution. We strongly encourage you to reflect on the content of this book, and the other leadership material you are no doubt absorbing, and begin to develop your own style of leadership — a style that works for you.

If we view leadership as an art, this book suggests how to paint a picture, but no one can paint for you. We have offered tools, but you will decide what picture you want to paint and how you want it to look. In this, leadership is not an exact science, it is an art individualized by leaders.

Second, we remind you that leadership is also a journey. The leader you are today is not, hopefully, the leader you will be tomorrow. Leaders are works in progress. All leaders stumble along the way, make bad calls and take actions that they later realize were not the best. But great leaders use their experiences — all their interpersonal and leadership experiences, successes and failures — as learning opportunities. Great leaders focus on continual growth.

As you progress through your leadership journey, we encourage you take focused steps to continually improve your practice of leadership as an art. Drawing on the work on building team mental models, we suggest leaders use a similar process to develop their own leadership mental model. That is, on a regular basis, leaders should assess what they are doing that works. Further, and perhaps more important, they assess their failures as well. They determine what they will do differently in the future and adjust their behaviors accordingly. This reflection and adjustment process is ongoing. It is the leader's journey.

----

1.   Hamel, G. & Valikanges, L. (2003). The quest for resilience. *Harvard Business Review, 81*(9), 52–65.

2.   Steiger, B. (2006). Special report, discouraged doctors: Survey results, doctors say morale is hurting. *Physician Executive, 32*(6), 6-15.

3.   Kornacki, M.J. & Silversin, J. (2012). *Leading Physicians Through Change: How to achieve and sustain results.* (2nd ed.). Tampa: FL: American College of Physicians Executives, p. x.

4.   Handy, C. (1995). *The Age of Paradox.* Boston: Harvard Business Review Press, p. 259.

5.   Brown, S.L.; Brown, R.M.; & Penner, L.A. (2011). *Moving Beyond Self-Interest: Perspectives from evolutionary biology, neuroscience, and the social sciences.* New York: Oxford University Press. Dutton, J.E.; Workman, K.M.; & Hardin, A.E. (2014). Compassion at work. *The Annual Review of Organizational Psychology and Organizational Behavior, 1,* 277-304.

6.   Armstrong, K. (2010). *Twelve Steps to a Compassionate Life.* New York: Anchor Books, p. 296.

7.   Ibid., p. 6.

8.   Avolio, B.J. & Gardner, W.L. (2005). Authentic leadership development: Getting to the root of positive forms of leadership. *The Leadership Quarterly, 16,* 315-338. Gentry, W.A.; Weber, T.J.; & Sadri, G. (2010). *Empathy in the Workplace: A tool for effective leadership.* Greensboro, NC: Center for Creative Leadership.

9.   Gentry, *et al.,* 2010.

10. Kanov, J.M.; Maitlis, S.; Worline, M.C.; Dutton, J.E.; Frost, P.J.; & Lilius, J.M. (2004). Compassion in organizational life. *American Behavioral Scientist, 47*(6), 808-827.

11. Ibid., p. 810.

CPSIA information can be obtained at www.ICGtesting.com
Printed in the USA
LVOW07s0501201015

458886LV00003B/4/P